£1.50

Day Surgery
Principles and Nursing Practice

No later ed 04/10

Day Surgery
Principles and Nursing Practice

Edited by

Heather Cahill
BSc (Hons), RGN, RMN, RCNT Cert Ed(Leeds)
Pathway Leader, Acute Care, Department of Health Studies, University of York

and

Ian Jackson
MB ChB(Aberdeen), FRCA
Head of Service, Anaesthetics, Theatre and Day Unit Services, York District Hospital

with contributions by

Terry Wilson
MEd, BA(Hons), Dip Nursing, RMN, RNT
Lecturer in Health Studies, Advanced Diploma in Counselling,
Department of Health Studies, University of York

Baillière Tindall
PUBLISHED IN ASSOCIATION WITH THE RCN
ROYAL COLLEGE OF NURSING

London Philadelphia Toronto Sydney Tokyo

Baillière Tindall 24–28 Oval Road
London NW1 7DX

The Curtis Center
Independence Square West
Philadelphia, PA 19106-3399, USA

Harcourt Brace & Company
55 Horner Avenue
Toronto, Ontario, M8Z 4X6, Canada

Harcourt Brace & Company, Australia
30–52 Smidmore Street
Marrickville
NSW 2204, Australia

Harcourt Brace & Company, Japan
Ichibancho Central Building
22-1 Ichibancho
Chiyoda-ku, Tokyo 102, Japan

This book is printed on acid-free paper

A catalogue record for this book is available from the British Library

ISBN 0-7020-2028-1

Typeset by Paston Press Ltd, Loddon, Norfolk
Printed and bound in Great Britain by The Bath Press, Bath

Contents

Preface

The last 10 years have witnessed a significant expansion in day surgery activity, and there is little doubt that these increases will continue as it offers many patients a cost effective, quality service without the need for an overnight stay. As both the number and the variety of procedures deemed suitable for day surgery increases so too do the needs and demands of patients, bringing the skills required of nurses working in the specialty to meet these demands clearly into focus.

Recognition of the likely potential for day surgery is reflected in the growth of post-registration educational opportunities for nurses in day surgery areas. Similarly, rightful emphasis is now being placed upon day surgery and its position at the interface between primary and secondary care in pre-registration nursing curricula. Busy, integrated day surgery units offer tremendous perioperative experience and a wealth of clinical learning opportunities for student nurses on Adult Branch programmes.

Our own experience of such developments in education and practice revealed to us the need for an in-depth textbook designed specifically for those nurses and other health care professionals working in day surgery. The book aims to equip nurses and other practitioners (through the promotion of reflection and exploration of relevant theory), with both knowledge and clinical skills in comprehensive patient assessment and perioperative management. We recognize the need for evidence-based practice and we therefore draw on contemporary research and literature in our discussion of a range of pertinent subjects. In writing the book, we hope to enhance the reader's awareness of the development of contemporary day surgery provision and invite them to assess the potential implications of emerging technology on their role and on the quality of patient care. 'Reflection points' throughout the text reinforce the analytical approach to clinical practice.

Although each chapter of the book covers a different topic and is therefore complete in itself, the sequence of the chapters, to some extent, follows a 'typical' patient's progression through the service. Firstly (in Chapters 1 and 2), we explore the factors influencing the development of day surgery services and some of the economic arguments surrounding its growth and popularity with Trusts in the UK. Chapter 3 examines the patient's recognition of symptoms, their decision to seek help and their initial consultation with their GP; patients' individual communication needs and the necessary skills required of nurses are explored in detail in Chapter 4. The safety and well-being of patients undergoing day surgery hinges on the vital processes of pre-admission assessment and selection and are the focus of Chapter 5, whilst theoretical frameworks for patient assessment, admission protocols and standards for care planning are addressed in Chapter 6.

The book promotes a 'perioperative' approach to patient management and nursing organization and development. Roles and practices in pre-operative preparation, anaesthesia, theatre, first-stage recovery and postoperative management are comprehensively explored in Chapters 7 to 11. Chapter 12 addresses the all important issues of quality and audit within the day surgery context, whilst in the last chapter we look to a possible future.

There are a great many people who have provided inspiration and encouragement to us both during this project and we gratefully acknowledge their input. Specifically, we would like to thank our respective partners, John and Susan, for their support, Kerry McKay and all the staff at York Day Surgery and Treatment Unit, as well as all ENB A21 students past and present at the University of York. Thanks are also due to Helen David, John Dean, Jacqueline Curthoys and especially to Terry Wilson, for his contribution of an excellent chapter on communication needs.

Heather Cahill and Ian Jackson
York 1997

Chapter 1 Day surgery – historical perspectives and current day provision

Overview

This chapter explains the history of early ambulation following surgery and shortened hospital stay and how this is critical to the future of day surgery. Socio-political trends over the past 20 years that have contributed to the development of day surgery are explored. Our aim is to provide the reader with a greater understanding of not only the rich background of research and expertise in this field but also of the degree of political interest generated by the potential for both health and economic gains. The various types of day surgery facilities are described with attention to their relative strengths and weaknesses. The development of day surgery in differing health care systems is also considered with particular emphasis on the useful experience gained in this field in the USA.

It is important that lessons from the past and the work of nursing and clinical pioneers are remembered to avoid trying to reinvent the wheel; many problems we now face have been solved previously, therefore we suggest that all readers take some time to read this chapter.

Chapter Focus

- Early developments
- Growth of day surgery in the UK
- The influence of the British Association of Day Surgery (BADS)
- The American experience
- European developments
- Facilities for day surgery

Introduction

No perspective on day surgery should ignore the change in medical and nursing thinking that was required to move from the ethos of the therapeutic importance of rest following surgery. From the late 1800s until the 1940s, rest was still seen as a major contribution to the recovery of patients following surgery (Hilton 1892). Indeed, bed rest for 2 weeks following major surgery was not unusual and many hospitals had separate convalescence units situated in the countryside or in sea resorts. However, in the post-war period there was a gradual increase in the number of publications supporting a reduction in not only the duration of bed rest but also the length of hospital stay (Leithauser 1946, Asher 1947). The move to early ambulation following surgery had started. The evidence of the benefits of early ambulation and indeed the dangers of prolonged bed rest gradually mounted (Blodgett & Beattie 1946, Palumbo *et al.* 1952). In the 1950s, the potential for early ambulation, shorter stay and indeed day surgery to provide economic advantages was first considered. Palumbo and colleagues mention the possibility of treating more patients through the same number of beds due to reduction in lengths of stay and Farquharson (1955) considered the potential impact for patients on waiting lists.

Even before this time, there were enthusiastic proponents of day surgery on both sides of the Atlantic. Nicholl (1909) reported his work on nearly 9000 children who underwent day surgery for such conditions as harelip, hernia, talipes and mastoid disease at the Royal Hospital for Sick Children in Glasgow. This was the work of a gifted enthusiast who was quite simply years ahead of his time. Ten years later in the USA, Waters (1919) reported on his 'Downtown Anesthesia Clinic' which provided care for dental and minor surgery cases. It is interesting to note that Nicholl showed his understanding of successful day surgery by stressing the importance of suitable home conditions and co-operation with general practitioners. These points were repeated nearly 50 years later by Farquharson and again currently in many articles about 'good practice' in day surgery.

The 1960s saw the development of one of the first stand-alone day surgery units within a hospital in the UK at the Hammersmith Hospital (Calnan & Martin 1971), though this had became an increasingly common facility in the USA during this period. The 1970s brought the first 'free standing' facilities – another concept that had been, and still is, very successful in the USA.

What Happened in the UK

The gradual move to day surgery in UK was largely being pushed by a few enthusiasts throughout the 1970s and 1980s until a report titled 'Guidelines for Day Case Surgery' was produced in 1985 (revised in 1992) by the Royal College of Surgeons of England. This report stated that 'day surgery is now considered the best option for fifty per cent of all patients undergoing elective procedures' and was published at a time when the national average was less than 15%.

Four years later the British Association of Day Surgery (BADS) was formed as a multi-disciplinary organization involving clinicians, nurses, operating department assistants (ODAs), managers and even architects. The common link was in their belief in day surgery and the potential advantages for patients and the National Health Service (NHS). They also recognized that to successfully increase levels of day surgery considerable attention had to be paid to quality.

The possibilities for day surgery were then recognized by two key reports. The first, published in 1989 by the NHS Management Executive's (NHSME's) Value for Money Unit (VFM) (known as the Bevan Report), supported the concept of day surgery and concluded that costs of treating patients as day cases were demonstrably less than treating them as inpatients. As this area was beyond the remit of this report a further detailed examination was commissioned by the VFM Unit which we cover later in the chapter. In 1990, the Audit Commission became responsible for the external audit of the NHS; this requires them to explore health topics with respect to economy, efficiency and effectiveness in the use of resources. Their first report, entitled 'A Short Cut To Better Services' examined day surgery in England and Wales. There is little doubt that this publication was a major catalyst for the development of day surgery provision within the UK and we suggest it is well worth reading. In the preface, the report argues that 'Day surgery has not expanded as fast as it might have done and performance varies considerably between health authorities.' The report introduces the concept of a 'basket' of 20 common procedures (accounting for 30% of all admissions in all surgical specialties) that could be performed as day surgery. The performance of 54 district health authorities in these 20 procedures was audited and when the results were compared the large variation became apparent. The largest variation was for carpal tunnel release with some districts performing them all as inpatients whilst others reported that they were all performed as day cases. The smallest variation was for repair of inguinal hernia but even here some units reported performing them all as inpatients whilst others performed 40% of them as day cases.

It was calculated in the report that if all units improved to the same performance as the top 25% for each procedure then 87 000 existing inpatients per year could be treated as day cases releasing £10 million which could then be used to treat an extra 98 000 day cases per year. The report went further as having found this variability in performance they state, 'The Commission therefore decided to identify the obstacles to growth and to suggest ways of overcoming them consistent with maintaining and improving standards of patient care'.

The report then goes on to consider six main barriers to change which included lack of specialist facilities, poor management of existing units and clinicians' preferences for more traditional approaches often backed up by a belief that patients do not like day surgery. Some possible solutions to these barriers are covered in considerable detail and the report ends with recommendations for hospitals, district health authorities (DHAs), regional health authorities, the Department of Health and the medical and nursing Royal Colleges.

The publication of this report was a major milestone in the development of day surgery in the UK and led to the publication of two further important documents the first of which signalled the political interest in this field.

'Day Surgery – Making it Happen' was published by the VFM Unit of the NHSME (1991). This report, though seeming to build on the lessons from the Audit Commission, was actually commissioned due to recommendations contained in the Bevan Report previously mentioned. Though it was very much concerned with good practice in the design and management of day units, their staffing and the management of issues such as quality and training, it also points out the potential financial gains for the NHS.

The next report of interest was a further publication by the Audit Commission in 1991 entitled 'Measuring Quality: The Patient's View of Day Surgery'. This introduced a questionnaire which allowed assessment of patients' perception of the day surgery services they received. With this the Audit Commission provided part of the answer to two of the barriers they had previously identified:

- the lack of information to assess current performance
- the belief of many clinicians that patients did not like day surgery.

The results of the use of the questionnaire in three health authorities were included in the publication and demonstrated that 80% of day case patients said they preferred being treated as a day case and that 83% said they would recommend it to a friend in a similar situation.

These reports all played a part in raising the level of knowledge and awareness about the potential for day surgery within the NHS and the government. The early 1990s saw the formation of regional 'task forces' to oversee the investment of considerable sums of money to promote day surgery. This led to the formation of many new day surgery units – another one of the barriers to change envisaged by the Audit Commission. A National Day Surgery Task Force was formed and this group successfully published a 'toolkit' which can be used by clinicians, nurses and managers as an aid to set up or review day surgery services (NHSME 1993).

It is evident that considerable encouragement was being given by the government via the NHSME, the Audit Commission and the regional health authorities at this time. Targets were set for increasing the level of day surgery to 50% of elective surgery by the year 2000 and support provided (financial and organizational advice) to help providers achieve this. What may be less apparent but should not be forgotten is the contribution of BADS and its members. Indeed, perusal of many of the reports mentioned above will reveal the involvement of key nursing, clinical and managerial representatives from the committee of this association. Their involvement demonstrates not only respect for these pioneers but also for this association. It should be noted that this group has grown to a membership of over 1000 in just 6 years.

The Current Position

Over the past 5 years, day surgery has grown from 15% to over 30% of elective surgery and now levels of day surgery for several operations form part of the assessment for the hospital league table system. The NHS Executive (previously the NHSME) has issued new advice on the levels that can be achieved. Following the success of provider hospitals in responding to the challenge and increasing their levels of day surgery we now use the term 'thresholds' rather than targets. The expectation is that 60% should be achieved by the 1996/97 financial year. The challenge is there and we as the providers of these services have to rise to this but at all times we must ensure this does not compromise quality for our patients. We make no apologies that this is a theme that the reader will find repeated throughout this book.

What Happened Elsewhere

Development of day surgery in the USA, Canada and Australia was at a much quicker pace than in the UK. The financial advantages were quickly seized upon, particularly in the largely private health care system found in the USA. Free-standing ambulatory surgery centres (ASCs) flourished in the 1970s but really became popular in the 1980s with changes in their recognition and reimbursement. In 1982, Medicare reimbursed about 100 procedures in free-standing ASCs but by 1991 this had increased to over 1200 procedures. The number of free-standing ASCs grew in parallel with this increase in potential income from 127 to 1221 over a similar period. By 1989, these were performing over 2 million procedures per year (Wolfson *et al.* 1993).

Over 60% of all elective operations are now performed as day case procedures in the USA with similar figures in Canada and Australia. The reason for the more rapid expansion in day surgery within these countries and the USA in particular is largely due to the desire of medical insurance companies to contain rising health care costs. However, variations in definitions of what is a day-case procedure should also be considered. In the USA, day surgery is defined as any procedure following which the patient is discharged within 24 h, somewhat different to the UK where patients are admitted and discharged within the working day. Perhaps 4-, 6- or 8-h surgery would be a more appropriate description for day surgery in the UK! Furthermore, it is difficult to compare statistics between countries as even definitions

Learning Points

The first Audit Commission report is helpful here as it classifies patients into three main categories: inpatients, outpatients and day cases:

- ***Inpatients*** – stay in hospital overnight
- ***Outpatients*** – come for minor procedures, investigations or consultations and leave as soon as they are over
- ***Day cases*** – do not stay in hospital overnight, but do need to stay for a short time after a procedure, for recovery.

of what is a day surgery procedure or an outpatient procedure vary tremendously. The reader should be aware that even within the UK this problem of definitions leads to variations in statistics recorded by hospitals and purchasers across the country. We deal with this important question of definition later in the chapter.

Most European countries are starting to become interested in day surgery but are some way behind the progress we have made in the UK. The large variation in day surgery levels and the low overall performance in these countries has much to do with the organization of their health services. A major example is Germany, where there are somewhat perverse incentives which make it financially rewarding to avoid performing day surgery. These issues are being brought to the surface and many countries are forming multidisciplinary day surgery groups similar to BADS which will push for the necessary changes. There are now both European and international associations being formed from members of these groups.

The report goes on to say, 'typically, day-case patients would stay in hospital for a morning or an afternoon. Exceptionally they might need to stay for a whole working day'. This deals with a broad definition for day cases but what of surgery? NHSME (1991) offers the following definition:

> An operation or procedure performed on a patient who is admitted on a non-residential basis. It will include minor and intermediate procedures carried out under local and general anaesthesia or sedation, for which a period of recovery is generally necessary, as well as procedures involving special equipment, such as endoscopies, where they are performed in operating theatres. The definition excludes, however, minor procedures which can be carried out on a day basis in A & E Departments and in Out-patients.

Finally, we include a more simple definition provided by the Royal College of Surgeons (1992):

> A surgical day case is a patient who is admitted for investigation or operation on a planned non-resident basis and who none the less requires facilities for recovery.

There are common threads throughout all these definitions and it is important to be aware of not only what is currently defined as day surgery by professional and government agencies but also the degree of latitude available in the interpretation of these. Some examples may be useful here to demonstrate this point:

- Reduction of nasal fractures was one of the Audit Commission's 'basket' of procedures and has been used as an example of a day surgery procedure. However, this procedure is performed in the outpatient department in many hospitals.
- Gastroscopy and colonoscopy are procedures often performed under sedation and the patient requires facilities for recovery – do we count these as day surgery patients?

Therefore, comparison of performance figures between hospitals, regions and between countries must be undertaken with an open mind to what is being counted.

Facilities for Day Surgery

There are several ways of providing day surgery services:

- self-contained day surgery unit – free-standing
- self-contained day surgery unit – integrated with main hospital
- self-contained day ward – using dedicated theatres in main theatre complex
- self-contained day ward – patients incorporated on inpatient theatre lists
- day patients admitted to any ward and patients incorporated on inpatient theatre lists.

The emphasis throughout the recent publications promoting day surgery mentioned earlier in this chapter has been on the efficiency of self-contained units and those with their own theatres in particular. Self-contained units integrated with the main hospital and self-contained day wards using dedicated theatres are the most common types of unit in this country. This compares with the USA where the free-standing and integrated day surgery units are more popular. These types of unit offer the most efficient use of resources by providing the best chance of maximizing throughput and minimizing the cost per patient. This is reflected in the USA by the lower charges of free-standing units compared to hospital-based units. The issues of costs, overheads and the economics of day surgery are covered in more detail in Chapter 2.

There are advantages and disadvantages with each type of service.

Free-standing

This type of unit brings advantages of reduced overheads in the USA but there are few free-standing units in the UK that are not owned by a Trust hospital and therefore have to take a share of all the Trust's overheads. Parking, a major problem in the UK, is usually not a problem. However, they bring problems that increase with the distance from their main supplier of medical and paramedical manpower. Support services from physiotherapy and laboratory services to intensive care and radiology are remote from the unit. Do outpatient clinics take place on site? If not, it means further trips for patients if pre-admission assessment is used. However, this may not necessarily be a bad thing (see Chapter 5). Travelling time of medical staff to and from the unit can be an inefficient use of a valuable resource. Admission of a patient to a hospital following problems as simple as unrelieved vomiting is also more difficult.

Integrated

This type of unit is seen by many as being ideal. Full support services are available and it is easy for patients to visit the unit on the same day as their outpatient clinic visit for pre-assessment. There is no loss of medical time due to travelling and if the unexpected happens, for example the patient requiring a laparotomy following failure to visualize the fallopian tubes during a sterilization, then it is easy to perform the procedure and then admit the patient.

Day Ward – Dedicated Theatre(s) in Main Theatre Complex

The distance between the ward area and the main theatre complex is important in this situation. The efficiency of day surgery depends on the rapid changeover of patients in theatre so that valuable theatre time is not lost. Therefore, efficient transfer of patients is important and becomes increasingly difficult with separation of the theatre and ward areas.

Day Ward – No Dedicated Theatres

This begins to not only reduce the efficiency of day surgery but can also have serious effects on the quality of service for day patients. It is inappropriate to fill up the occasional half hour on the end of a list to perform day surgery as these cases should be done early on the list to ensure maximal time for recovery. The risk of cancellation is also high if patients are following a large case. Putting day patients on the beginning of the list is more satisfactory but can also lead to the problem of lists over running their allotted time – a problem all too familiar to those with theatre experience. However they are managed, the tendency is for the day cases not to receive the degree of attention they require. The anxiety felt by these unpremedicated patients is not helped by transfer to a busy, threatening main theatre complex.

Day Patients Admitted to Inpatient Wards – No Dedicated Theatres

This was the situation to be found in most hospitals 5–10 years ago. Perhaps the only advantage offered by this system is the avoidance of the non-recurring capital outlay required to develop a day surgery unit. The disadvantages are many and include poor utilization; no reduction in costs by transferring to day surgery as inpatient bed numbers have to be maintained; and problems admitting scheduled patients due to beds being filled with emergency admissions. More importantly, quality for the patient suffers as the nursing staff are busy looking after the major surgical cases returned from theatre and the acutely ill emergency admissions and so have little time for day cases undergoing 'minor' procedures. This is not the fault of these staff but more of a reflection of the prioritization necessary when workload is high.

Summary

History has shown us that day surgery is not new. Many important lessons have already been learnt and should not be forgotten. Development of day surgery in Australia, Canada and the USA has been much quicker and this reflects the financial incentives in these countries. What qualifies as a day surgery procedure is variable across the globe. This variation is also apparent within the UK as there are large differences between regions and even between local hospitals in the same region.

We have considered the reasons for the fundamental differences in design of day surgery units between the USA and the UK. How the design of a day surgery facility can effect not only the efficiency of the unit but also the quality of service has also been reviewed.

Key Points

- Early pioneers of day surgery include Nicholl from Glasgow who reported his work in 1909.
- The importance of social circumstances and co-operation with general practitioners was reported by Nicholl in 1909 and repeated in the work of Farquharson in 1955.
- The possibility of treating more patients through less beds and the impact this may have on waiting lists was described in the 1950s.
- Development of day surgery in the UK is due to the combined efforts of managers, nurses, clinicians, BADS and the government.
- Definitions of what is day surgery change not only throughout the world but also between regions and even hospitals in the UK.

Recommended Reading

Audit Commission (1990) **A short cut to better services: Day surgery in England and Wales.** London: HMSO.

References

Asher, R. A. J. (1947) **The dangers of going to bed.** *British Medical Journal* **ii**: 967–968.

Audit Commission (1990) **A short cut to better services: Day surgery in England and Wales.** London: HMSO.

Audit Commission (1991) **Measuring quality: The patient's view of day surgery.** NHS Occasional Papers. London: HMSO.

Blodgett, J. B. and Beattie, E. J. (1946) **Early post operative rising: a statistical study of post operative complications.** *Surgery, Gynaecology and Obstetrics* **82**: 485.

Calnan, J. and Martin, P. (1971) **Development and practice of an autonomous minor surgery unit in a general hospital.** *British Medical Journal* **iv**: 92.

Farquharson, E. L. (1955) **Early ambulation with special references to herniorraphy as an outpatient procedure.** *Lancet* **ii**: 517–519.

Hilton, J. (1892) **Rest and Pain.** London: George Bell.

Leithauser, L. (1946) **Early Ambulation and Related Procedures in Surgical Management.** Oxford: Blackwell Scientific Publications.

NHSME (1993) **Day surgery – Report by the day surgery task force.** Heywood. BAPS Health Publication Unit.

NHSME VFM Unit (1991) **Day surgery – Making it happen.** London: HMSO.

NHSME VFM Unit (Bevan Report) (1989) **A study of the management and utilisation of operating departments.** London: HMSO.

Nicholl, J. H. (1909) **The surgery of infancy.** *British Medical Journal* **ii**: 753–756.

Palumbo, L. T., Paul, R. E. and Emery, F. B. (1952) **Results of primary inguinal hernioplasty.** *Archives of Surgery* **64**: 384–394.

Royal College of Surgeons of England (1992) **Report of the working party on guidelines for day case surgery** (Revised Edition). London: RCoS.

Waters, R. M. (1919) **The down-town anesthesia clinic.** *American Journal of Surgery* **33**(Suppl): 71–73.

Wolfson, J., Walker, G. and Levin, P. J. (1993) **Free-standing ambulatory surgery: Cost-containment winner?** *Healthcare Financial Management* **July**: 27–32.

Chapter 2 Economic factors and quality control in day surgery provision

Overview

This short chapter provides an basic introduction to the field of health care economics and some of the key terminology. We present a summary of the economic aspects of reports on day surgery including those from the Audit Commission and the NHS Executive and the financial benefits of day surgery are explored with particular attention to the maintenance of quality for both inpatient and day surgery patients. The chapter aims to encourage the reader to develop a critical approach to claims about cost savings and potential reduction in waiting lists.

Chapter Focus

- Terminology of health economics
- Issues in costing a service
- Reported savings in day surgery
- Problems arising in the assessment of savings

Introduction

This chapter was one of the most difficult for us to write as economics can quickly be turned into something that is both boring and incomprehensible. This is perhaps a reflection of the language of economics rather than the use of difficult concepts. In fact, we all have to balance our books (admittedly some better than others), deal with what we can or cannot afford this month (using cash, credit cards, hire purchase or leasing), consider the effects of interest rates on our mortgage or perhaps, if we are lucky, consider in which account to keep our money to obtain the best rate of return. Economics is a part of everyday life and we try to introduce some of the language and concepts of this subject whilst working through a comparison of costing between inpatient and day surgery. We consider why there should theoretically be a difference in the total costs involved and perhaps why these calculated savings are difficult to achieve.

In economic and structural terms, health care delivery comprises inputs, process and outputs. Figure 2.1 demonstrates the relationships.

Three terms appearing in this and other texts considering the economics of health care are 'economy', 'efficiency' and 'effectiveness'. First, let us be clear about what we mean by each of these terms:

- *Economy* is a term with which we all are familiar! In this context it means paying less for the same *input.*
- *Efficiency* is achieved either by reducing input whilst maintaining output, or increasing output with no increase in input; a measure of 'doing things right' (Jones & McDonnell 1993).

Figure 2.1 Operating structure of health care (adapted from Jones & McDonnell 1993)

Inputs (quite variable – combine to produce the processes of health care)
Financial resources
Material resources
Human resources
Information
Patients
Legal, fiscal and regulatory controls
↓
Process (activities that ensure economic use of resources takes place)
Organizational structure
Models/protocols of care
Resource allocation and utilization
Flow of activities
Monitoring and control mechanisms
↓
Output (relates to effectiveness and efficiency of resource use)
Throughput of services – number of discharges, number of deaths, etc.
Delivery of contracts
↓
Outcome (an evaluation of output)
Appropriateness and acceptability
Degree of health gain
Patient satisfaction
Value for money (VFM)

- *Effectiveness* is 'a measure of how successfully or otherwise, activities are being carried out' (Jones & McDonnell 1993); it is concerned with doing the 'right things' and that relates to both output and outcome.

Any potential savings from a move to day surgery would represent an *economy*; however, an increase in activity (which may reduce waiting lists) for the same money would represent an increase in *efficiency*. But according to Culyer (1991) there are a number of different types of efficiency, which include:

- the provision of only those services of which there is clear evidence of improved patient outcome – i.e. those that are *effective*
- provision of such effective services at minimum cost
- concentration of resources on effective services delivered at minimum cost to maximum patient benefit
- providing these services on such a scale that patient benefit outweighs additional costs.

It is possible therefore for a medical procedure to be effective but not efficient. If we ensure that *only* patients who were suitable for day surgery who attended our day unit then this would be *effective*. To consider the potential for day surgery to provide economy or efficiency savings we must consider the costs involved in the management of patients. This is not a simple procedure as historically in the health service there has been no need to cost procedures; furthermore, there are several different types of costs we must understand to gain a full picture.

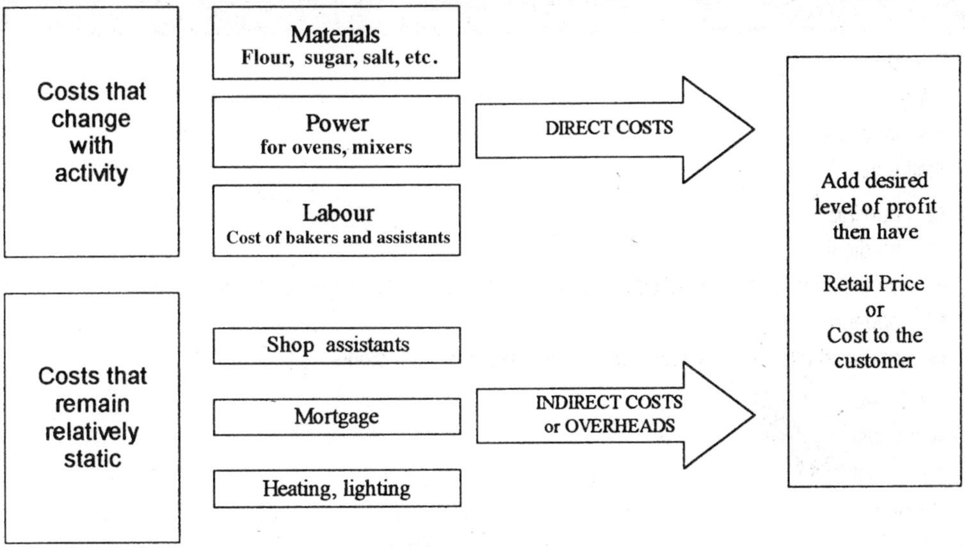

Figure 2.2 Costs incurred in a typical business

Let us first consider the types of costs involved in a simple business that consists of a combined bakery and shop unit (Fig. 2.2).

You will notice that costs are classified in two groups – *direct* and *indirect*. Direct costs are the costs of labour and materials that can be identified as relating directly to the product or service. In the above example the ingredients, cost of heating the ovens, and the cost of the labour in the bakery are *direct costs*. A feature of direct costs is that they increase as activity is increased, for example number of loaves of bread produced.

It will not surprise you to find that those costs not directly linked to the production of the bread are termed indirect costs, these being all the costs incurred in running an organization other than the direct costs. These are also sometimes called the *overheads*. Therefore the cost of heating and lighting the bakery and shop, the cost of the mortgage on the property and the salary of the sales assistants are all *indirect costs* or overheads. It can be seen that these remain stable to a degree with changing production in the bakery. However, if we continue to increase production there will come a certain point where we may have an increase in overheads due to the requirement for new sales staff, or a larger property.

Now we shall consider the costs associated with a patient coming into hospital for an operative procedure such as a hernia repair.

The list in Box 2.1, though extensive, is incomplete and many of you will think of costs that should be added; however, it will make a good starting point. Already you will have perhaps noted that some of the costs incurred are directly due to the procedure to be performed, for example the cost of the theatre time, the cost of the nursing staff, surgeon and anaesthetist for the operation, the cost of any sutures and dressings used, etc.

Box 2.2 shows a breakdown of some of the direct costs for our chosen procedure.

The indirect costs include such things as the cost of the managers in charge of the theatre and ward areas, as they do not directly look after the patient during their stay, the cost of the phone system, heating and lighting. Box 2.3 provides a more extensive list.

Therefore, it will be apparent that we cannot just consider the direct costs of an operation and hospital stay when we are working out how much we should charge the purchaser (general

Box 2.1 Costs linked to hospital admission for an operation

Dressings
Drugs
Theatre costs
Staff time

- nursing
- medical
- professions allied to medicine, e.g. physiotherapy, radiographers, laboratory staff
- portering
- administration, e.g. secretaries, medical records staff, clerks

Food
Ward costs
X-ray costs
Heating
Laundry
Lighting
Administration
Telephone

Box 2.2 Direct costs

Sending for patient
Cost of paper, postage

During patient stay
Ward costs – nursing and medical staff time, cost of drugs prescribed
Theatre costs – nursing and medical staff time, materials and drugs used

Following discharge
Community nurse follow-up, suture removal

practitioner or health authority). Each hospital has to also recoup the costs of their overheads and does this by allocating a proportion of these indirect costs to the price of each procedure or admission to the hospital.

Naturally, this is a gross oversimplification of what happens in the National Health Service (NHS) but it does provide an initial insight into the complications faced by those responsible for setting prices in our hospitals. It also begins to throw up a dilemma for hospitals if they move successfully to day surgery then a certain number of staff who previously were directly involved in the management of these patients are no longer involved – do they become an overhead (so the cost to the purchaser does not reduce) or are they removed (economy for the purchaser). Now we can consider how a move to day surgery may have an effect on *economy* or *efficiency*.

Box 2.3 Indirect costs (overheads)

Staff

- The chief executive and managerial staff
- senior nursing managers
- Nurse tutors
- Professions allied to medicine, e.g. physiotherapy, radiographers, laboratory staff
- Pharmacy staff
- Portering of samples, results, internal mail
- Administration, e.g. secretaries, medical records staff, clerks
- Domestics
- Hospital support services, e.g. plumbers, electricians, electronics
- Chaplain

Heating
Laundry
Maintenance
Estate management
Lighting
Administration
Telephone
Printing and stationery
Rates, rents, capital charges

Economy and Efficiency in Day Surgery – the Argument

The original Audit Commission report on day surgery (A Short Cut To Better Services) covered both these stating that 'day surgery offers two considerable advantages:

1. the service offered to patients can be better organized and suited to their needs, and above all can be provided sooner as faster throughput allows waiting lists to be reduced
2. hospital costs are lower and there is no evidence of significant offsetting cost increases for community support or extra care of patients at home.

Evidence quoted in support of these claims included two key references. First there was the Royal College of Surgeons of England (Guidelines for Day Case Surgery) and an extensive review (Morgan & Beech 1990) which demonstrated that day case surgery costs 40–50% less. However, the report goes on to warn that the calculations in these reports were based on studies of costs in the 1970s and that a more realistic estimate of savings may be around 25–30%. The crux of this potential saving then follows with the statement that 'the majority of the difference in hospital costs reflect differences in the "hotel" element (principally nursing and catering costs …'. Therefore to make these savings, levels of nursing and support staff must be reduced. This implies the closure of beds and even wards – this is covered in more detail later in the chapter.

The Bevan Report in 1989 suggested that the average cost of a day theatre was 29% less than a theatre dealing with inpatients; however, the major reduction in costs in this report was again due to staff reductions made possible by the extensive use of local anaesthesia. In this case the reduction was primarily in medical staff – anaesthetists in particular. The private health insurers have contributed to the debate with the British United Provident Association (BUPA) publishing that the cost of day surgery procedures was 38% less than the average inpatient cost for the same procedure (Wiggins 1991).

The Royal College of Surgeons of England updated its earlier report in 1992 in which it devoted an interesting new section on the 'Economics of Day Surgery'. This section written by a member of the original Audit Commission team represents a landmark in a move to more realistic expectations of the potential savings that may be obtained by a move from inpatient surgery to day surgery. This is a valuable article which starts by providing a table of many of the articles published about the potential savings to be gained from a move to day surgery and the method used to calculate the saving. The article goes on to state that

> it is misleading to interpret differences in average costs as measures of the savings which might result from a substitution of day surgery for inpatient surgery. They are likely to be overestimates. The resource implications of more day surgery should be estimated directly by looking at precisely what changes are planned to take place.

Thus each hospital must look at its plan for implementing a transfer to day surgery. Indeed one report (Beech & Larkinson 1990) has stated that if the transfer does not result in the closure of a ward (and thus a reduction in staff) then the savings for a hospital may be as little as £6 per patient.

This last study demonstrated that efficiency improvements (i.e. using the resource released to treat more patients, rather than economy improvements, i.e. closing wards) would result in a much larger gain for an organization. It is interesting to note that support for the efficiency improvement stems back to original papers by Palumbo *et al.* (1952) who mention the possibility of treating more patients through the same number of beds and also Farquharson (1955) who considers the potential for day surgery to reduce waiting lists. It would appear that our problems have been faced before and indeed the same solutions considered!

Thus a move to day surgery can lead to economy or efficiency gains. The main point to remember is that to provide economy savings then a move to day surgery must result in cheaper prices to the purchaser. This in turn can only be achieved by reducing the direct costs of the organization (as can be produced in a day unit) whilst maintaining or reducing the indirect costs or overheads of the organization. Thus, to achieve economy gains the transfer of activity to day surgery must result in closure of sufficient number of beds to remove a ward and the equivalent number of staff. Staff represent the largest cost to the organization. The path to efficiency gains can be more attractive for an organization as it:

- provides the opportunity to treat more patients with
- potential reduction in waiting lists – thus improve position on national league tables
- avoids redundancy and improves morale.

However, we still have not explored all the possible costs involved in day surgery. Providing a quality service for patients is critical to the success of day surgery in any unit. Part of this quality is achieved by preventing the patient feeling that their visit was rushed and that the staff had no time to look after them. In a day surgery unit the staff have to deal with the total care of patients compressed into a few hours instead of several days. This care must include:

- welcoming patients to the unit
- explaining what is going to happen to both patients and carers
- making arrangements with carers for their return to pick up patients
- providing support prior to theatre
- ensuring patients are ready for theatre – consent, markings, safety issues
- caring for patients postoperatively – fluids, ensuring comfort, mobilization
- providing information to patients and their carers about postoperative instructions and what to expect
- ensuring patients are ready for discharge.

These are just a few vital areas for staff on a day unit; the important point here is that they take time and that is a scarce resource in day surgery. Additionally, there are other demands for nursing time in day surgery – one of the largest of these is pre-assessment of patients (see Chapter 5). Therefore, we must ensure that we have sufficient numbers of staff in our day wards to provide these services. This increases the cost of day surgery and may well have been ignored by many researchers in this field. We must ensure that patients do not receive a substandard service in the thrust towards providing more economical or efficient health care.

It is not yet safe to believe that we have considered all the costs of a move to day surgery. We must now consider the cost of removing the 'well and fit' patients from inpatient wards. What effect does this have on inpatient wards? Clearly, the removal of large numbers of what were fit patients using the ward mainly as a hotel facility and making relatively few demands on the ward staff will have an effect on the running of acute wards. When this occurs in conjunction with no reduction in occupancy levels of the ward (a situation that will arise if surgical beds are closed elsewhere or if the empty beds are used to treat more patients, i.e. an increase in surgical activity) then the dependency of the patients increases. The beds are occupied by people undergoing more complex surgery or are assessed as being unfit for day surgery; both these groups require more nursing care. If no further nursing resource is put into the ward then the level of service or quality of service it is possible for the nursing staff to provide is compromised. Once again, this is a feature of the move to day surgery that is not considered by most reviews into the economics of day surgery.

Summary

In this chapter we have considered some of the economic arguments surrounding day surgery. We have attempted to provide an introduction to some basic concepts such as direct and indirect costs and the system within the NHS of sharing these across an organization. Readers interested in this area should contact their local management accountant for further details of what is happening in their own hospital. In our experience these individuals are not only delighted to help interested staff but are also very capable of explaining the intricacies of a complex subject.

When reading articles about the potential 'cost savings' made possible by a move to day surgery it is important to reflect on whether the authors have considered the costs of appropriate levels of staffing in the day unit and on inpatient wards.

Key Points

- Economy is the concept of paying less for the same input.
- Efficiency is reducing input whilst maintaining output, or increasing output for the same input.
- Effectiveness is a measure of doing the 'right things'.
- Direct costs are the costs of labour and materials that can be identified as relating directly to a product or service.
- Indirect costs (or overheads) are all the costs incurred in running an organization other than the direct costs.
- The potential savings found in a move to day surgery have been over exaggerated in the past.
- Savings require the closure of wards and loss of staff.

Recommended Reading

Jones, A. and McDonnell, U. (1993) **Managing the Clinical Resource. An action-guide for health care professionals.** London: Baillière Tindall

A very clear and readable text; we particularly recommend chapters 1, 2 and 7

References

Audit Commission (1990) **A short cut to better services: Day surgery in England and Wales.** London: HMSO.

Beech, R. and Larkinson, J. (1990) **Estimating the financial saving from maintaining the level of acute services with fewer hospital beds.** *International Journal of Health Planning and Management* **5**: 89–103.

Culyer, A. (1991) **The promise of a reformed NHS: an economist's angle.** *British Medical Journal* **302**: 1253–1256.

Farquharson, E. L. (1955) **Early ambulation with special references to herniorraphy as an outpatient procedure.** *Lancet* **ii**: 517–519.

Jones, A. and McDonnell, U. (1993) **Managing the Clinical Resource. An action-guide for health care professionals.** London: Baillière Tindall.

Morgan, M. and Beech, R. (1990) **Variations in lengths of stay and rates of day case surgery: implications for the efficiency of surgical management.** *Journal of Epidemiology and Community Health* **44**: 90–105.

NHSME VFM Unit (Bevan Report) (1989) **A study of the management and utilisation of operating departments.** London: HMSO.

Palumbo, L. T., Paul, R. E. and Emery, F. B. (1952) **Results of primary inguinal hernioplasty.** *Archives of Surgery* **64**: 384–394.

Royal College of Surgeons of England (1992) **Report of the working party on guidelines for day case surgery** (Revised Edition). London: RCoS.

Wiggins, J. (1991) **The insurer's perspective on ambulatory surgery.** First European Congress on Ambulatory Surgery, Brussels, March: ABS 056.

Chapter 3 Patients' health beliefs, understanding of illness and expectations of health service provision

Overview

In this chapter we begin to focus our attention on the people who are the major consumers of day surgery services – the patients. In an attempt to more fully understand the people in our care, the chapter reviews some of the factors that influence their decisions to consult a doctor. We also explore the beliefs and values underlying these decisions and how, or indeed if, they relate to health behaviour and compliance with treatment.

An important element of recent health service reform has been the increased emphasis on patients' rights, choices and involvement in decision making regarding their care. Using self-care theory as a basis for discussion, the chapter also explores the extent to which patients expect or even desire this type of relationship with health professionals.

Chapter Focus

- Health, illness and illness behaviour
- Lay beliefs
- Lay referral and sectors of health care
- Patterns of consultation
- Predicting behaviour & compliance
- Patients expectations

Introduction

It is not surprising that for many nurses the path that patients follow to the day surgery unit only begins in the car park. Although consideration is generally given to patients' immediate feelings and concerns during the admission process, few nurses would concern themselves with how and why their patients made the decision to seek medical attention in the first instance. First, there is not enough time and second, it is arguable whether such an exploration would improve the patients' care during their stay. We are not therefore suggesting that nurses spend time eliciting such information. However, having a greater awareness of how individual's react and respond to symptoms, how they negotiate consultations with general practitioners and surgeons, and how they respond to prescribed treatments may indeed help to increase nurses' understanding of patients' differing reactions to the experience of day surgery. Understanding and acceptance of these lay beliefs is also fundamental to effective and meaningful health education, and there is little doubt that nurses in day surgery have an important role to play in this area, especially in small group and individual situations.

Illness and Illness Behaviour

> Once the economic barrier to health care had been removed with the setting up of the National Health Service, it was assumed that all those in need of medical care would consult their doctor or other appropriate medical services. No one questioned whether an individual would be able to know whether he or she needed medical attention or not. (Morgan, Calnan & Manning 1985)

Repeated studies of illness rates and illness behaviour continually demonstrate that whilst high levels of ill health exist throughout the community, only a fraction of the symptoms suffered result in medical consultation (Morgan *et al.* 1985). According to Scambler and Scambler (1984), as few as one in 18 symptom episodes are ever referred to a general practitioner, and Mechanic (1968) demonstrates that people with the same symptoms show very different rates of consultation. Whilst it is safe to assume that most of these symptoms are mild and readily dealt with without the need for medical assistance (think about what you did the last time you had a sore throat, or a headcold), it is also clear that other more serious symptoms continue to go undiagnosed and untreated. Many sociologists have referred to this phenomenon as an 'illness iceberg' (Scambler & Scambler 1984, Morgan *et al.* 1985, Hannay 1988, Armstrong 1989), with doctors, both in hospital and general practice, only seeing its very tip. The presence of this iceberg indicates that many other non-medical factors help to influence how people perceive, interpret and act upon their symptoms. Not least of these factors is the priority that health or illness has in the life of any individual.

Day surgery today is a high-profile service, frequently under the public gaze, and promoted as the cost-effective way of meeting purchaser needs for up to 50% of all elective surgery (Royal College of Surgeons 1992). Nurses working in this speciality are quickly socialized into a kind of 'acute sector culture' with an understandable emphasis on effectiveness and efficiency in a climate of ever-limited resources. Perhaps it is too easy for them to accept some of the values and beliefs inherent in that culture, but these are values and beliefs that their patients, as likely as not, do not share. For example, witness the undisguised frustration and irritation associated with patients arriving late, or even worse, failing to attend for clinic appointments, investigations and surgery. This form of 'non-compliance' clearly exasperates health care professionals and unfortunately results in such patients being labelled difficult or irresponsible. The phrase 'they are wasting our valuable time' is too frequently heard, and is often followed up by angry letters to general practitioners.

Yet these 'did not attend' (DNA) rates cannot simply reflect widespread foolhardiness and lack of responsibility on behalf of the public, as is the prevailing professional view. It is indeed far more likely that on the day, other priorities needed attention, for example their child's school play or a helping a friend, or it may be that they simply did not have enough money for the bus to hospital.

As differences in opinion on health and illness and their priorities often exist between members of different professional groups (e.g. doctors and nurses), so too they exist between professional groups and the general public. There is still a pervasive tendency amongst health professionals to define health largely in physical terms, placing considerable emphasis on what McQueen (cited by Dines 1994) refers to as the 'holy four': exercise, alcohol consumption, smoking and diet. Whilst there is little doubt that many members of the public now have more knowledge and understanding of health matters, and in particular the role of these lifestyle behaviours, such emphasis simply perpetuates the medical model of health (i.e. freedom from medically defined

Reflection Points

- How are patients who fail to attend for appointments dealt with in your area?
- How would you describe the attitudes of your colleagues and clinicians towards those who do not attend?

disease). The practice also tends to devalue the equally significant mental, social, emotional and spiritual dimensions of health, whilst at the same time distancing the professionals from the people they are caring for. A nurse who believes that health is defined as having a normal blood pressure and being the correct weight for height will, not surprisingly, communicate these beliefs in any health education he or she may undertake. But such health education will have little meaning for the individual who thinks of health more in terms of feeling at peace, or simply having enough strength to get through the day.

Symptoms, which to the professional are clear indicators of disease that may need urgent treatment, first need to be interpreted by the lay person within their own frame of reference. Similarly, symptoms viewed as signs of illness in one society are not necessarily seen as such in another; ill health is clearly defined by cultural values and social norms. Mechanic (1968) outlines a number of factors that he believes to be commonly associated with seeking help. These include the perceived seriousness of the symptoms, their visibility and meaning, the extent to which the symptoms interfere with normal activities and their frequency and persistence. So although the subsequent course of action would be relatively clear-cut to the clinician on recognition of a group of symptoms, the lay person does not necessarily interpret their symptoms in that way.

Studies of illness behaviour suggest that it is important to separate the concept of *disease* from that of *illness*. Helman (1990) defines disease as something that affects an organ, and illness as something that affects a person. He also refers to Cassell's witty but accurate observation that illness is what a person feels on the way to the doctor's surgery, but disease is what they have on the way home. Helman sees illness as a subjective response, both of the individual and those around them to their being unwell; it includes not only the actual *experience* of ill-health, but also, and possibly more importantly, the *meaning* given to that experience. These sophisticated lay interpretations are influenced by individual personality and emotional factors, in addition to the wider cultural and socio-economic context in which they occur (Helman 1990). Therefore, the decision to consult a doctor represents only one of a number of possible courses of action. The concern amongst clinicians about the failure of people to consult initiated considerable research into lay theories of health, illness and illness behaviour. Calnan (1987) suggests that it soon became clear to health professionals that it was probably better to try and find out *how* people come to feel ill, and what they do about it, rather than continually asking why they do not use official health services.

Research into Lay Beliefs

This short review does not attempt to include all the valuable work done in this area. For those new to this subject, and wish to know more, we would direct you to the original sources included in the reference section.

Ideas about health and illness vary between societies, between different groups in the same society and within the same society over time. Thus, illness behaviour (the response to illness and the tendency or reluctance to define any symptom as a health problem and seek medical care) varies between cultural and social groups. That said, the first thing that becomes apparent is the number of similarities that exist between the studies that explore lay theories of health and illness. One of the earliest was the seminal work of Claudine Herzlich (1973) in France. She carried out in-depth interviews with 80 predominantly middle-class individuals from Paris and Normandy. Analysis of their accounts revealed three different dimensions of health. First, health was described as a positive state, a state of not being ill. Herzlich classified this as health *in a vacuum*. The second classification was health as a reserve, a resistance to illness; a state to be had and to be held on to. Finally, health was described as a state of equilibrium, which allows for full realization of health reserve. Importantly, Herzlich's participants saw health as an *internal* state; that is, generated by the individual. They believed that temperament and hereditary factors were important contributors to their health and they also attached moral associations to it; there was almost an obligation or duty to be healthy. On the other hand, these individuals viewed illness as a phenomenon with an *external* cause; a result of urban life, and therefore largely out of their control. Similar findings were reported by Pill and Stott (1982) in Cardiff. They interviewed 41 mothers with small children from social class IV or V, and again three broad dimensions of health were identified. Health was described as:

- the absence of illness
- the capacity to function as expected and to be able to cope
- being cheerful, enthusiastic and effervescent.

About 50% of those interviewed in this study were quite fatalistic in their views about the causes of disease and furthermore, appeared resistant to changing these views. Later research by these same authors with some 200 women from the same social groups revealed that 'practically everyone accepts the reality of illness caused by factors outside individual control, while a smaller proportion *also* accept that individual action can contribute to the likelihood of falling ill' (Pill & Stott 1985).

Blaxter and Paterson (1982) also studied socially disadvantaged families; this time the respondents being mothers and daughters. The findings once more were similar, but these women's definitions of health were even more functional, in that health was more likely to be defined as functional fitness to contend with difficulties and carry out normal roles. Analysis of their accounts once more revealed health and illness as moral categories, with an implicit recognition of a duty to be healthy. Normalization and accommodation of what they defined as 'normal illnesses' into everyday life were a common feature of these accounts. Morgan *et al.* (1985) suggest this accommodation is one reason why people in more disadvantaged circumstances participate considerably less in preventative health programmes. They go on to state that these views 'are clearly influenced by the experience of a high prevalence of ill-health in this group'.

Rory Williams' (1983) study of the elderly in Aberdeen identified a classification of health that almost mirrors that of Herzlich. These 70 respondents seemed to see health as something internal and positive, defined in terms of integrity, inner strength and the ability to contend with difficulties. If these qualities or attributes were intact, then they perceived themselves as

Box 3.1 Case study

Cervical cancer causes the death of approximately 2000 women annually in the UK, although wide variations exist between the social classes, with six times more deaths in women in Social Class V than in Social Class I (Davies 1991). But it would be wrong to assume that all women in the lower social groups share similar experiences of health and illness; repeated evidence also suggests that inequalities in health exist *within* social groups (Whitehead 1988). Although there were nearly 5 million smears carried out in 1987, representing an increase of 62% since 1976, we also know that 80% of women who have invasive cervical cancer have *never* had a smear (Jacobson *et al.* 1991). Also, whilst death rates for the disease have remained relatively constant, and mortality amongst women in the 45–64 years age group has fallen since the early 1980s, there has been a slight increase in rates amongst women aged 25–44.

Overall, and despite the 25 years of the screening programme, the incidence and mortality from the disease has not reduced significantly. Elkind *et al.* (1989) identify inaccessibility, failed communication and refusal amongst a number of barriers contributing to women in social classes IV and V's poor attendance for cervical screening. Martin and Main (1992) ascribe the term *refusal* to those women who have 'no *valid* reason to believe the test is inappropriate but who decide not to attend' (our emphasis). But from what we have seen, what constitutes a 'valid' reason? These authors seem to believe that practical issues around the venue of clinics, timing of appointments and fear and embarrassment of being tested are in some way *invalid*. Whilst we would not argue that a vital part of health education is to try and correct sensitively any erroneous beliefs, it is still important to accept these issues as valid within lay interpretations. The challenge for health educators is to provide value-free and straightforward information that not only accurately informs women of the function and value of the screening programme, but also explicitly acknowledges the importance of their own beliefs. Jacobson *et al.* (1991) argue that measures to increase acceptance of the smear test should be a primary objective for health authorities. Similar concerns are voiced about poor attendance for initial and repeat colposcopy, a common investigation carried out on day surgery units. These women are often thought careless and irresponsible by clinicians and nurses alike, but is this the case?

healthy, even in the presence of serious disease. Illness, on the other hand, was due to external factors in the environment and was deemed negative. As Dines (1994) points out, these findings indicate that those known to be more at risk of developing serious disease do not believe that individual action is of any use in their prevention. This constitutes a major challenge for those involved in health education and health promotion; the incidence of cervical cancer (outlined in Box 3.1) and the poor uptake of screening amongst those considered most at risk, provides a lucid example of such a challenge.

Generally, the young and the more affluent respondents in all of these studies felt that they had more control over their health and illness experiences than older people and those worse off financially. The younger groups placed more emphasis on the role of viruses, germs and social stressors than they did any lack of moral fibre in the causes of disease (Cornwell 1984). Also, parents demonstrated a strong moral obligation and responsibility towards their children's well-being, opting for a 'better to be safe than sorry' approach in the presence of symptoms. It is not surprising that parents are more likely to report symptoms in their child to their general practitioner than they would the same symptoms in themselves. Early referral for day or inpatient surgery is therefore much more common, as is early reporting of postoperative difficulties, problems that ironically many nurses and clinicians would perceive as trivial!

The findings of these studies, whilst showing how lay beliefs change across generations, still suggest that respondents' understandings of health, illness and disease are closely linked to their socio-economic circumstances. Only Calnan's (1987) comparative study of women from across all social groups failed to make a clear association between social class and definitions of health.

It is also of note that women are the focus of the majority of these studies, which raises some important concerns with regard to their methodologies and conclusions. Nathanson (1977) estimates that around 80% of respondents in interviews are women. Therefore, if women are frequently targeted in health surveys, more likely to respond than their partners and underreport symptoms in their partners (Clarke 1983), it follows that there will be an overall excess of self-reported illness in women. More recently, Backett (1990, 1991) has adopted a different approach, focusing on 28 families in *non-manual* occupations, and interviewing both men and women. The research also attempted to elicit the health beliefs of 52 children aged 4–12 years from these same families (which is nothing short of a methodological nightmare!). Interestingly, Backett's findings suggest that even in socially advantaged groups, there is still a large gap between what is understood and voiced about health and what is actually practised. Similar conclusions are drawn in the Health and Lifestyles Survey (Blaxter 1990); even if individuals hold positive values and accurate beliefs, there are as many barriers that intervene between intention and action as there are facilitators. This again challenges the commonly held assumption that it is only those in lower social groups that need health messages reinforced.

The notion of individuals carrying out activities which contribute to the maintenance of their health has been around in nursing for some time. Familiarized by Orem (1985), the idea is also recognized by a number of theorists as what people actually do, to a greater or lesser extent. Self-care is an important theme in the field of health promotion (Pender 1987). The fact that people want to be in charge of their own lives, look after themselves and make their own decisions is not in doubt; indeed it is heavily promoted by present government policies (Naidoo & Wills 1994). But some of the activities performed are potentially damaging to health, for example smoking and drinking alcohol, whilst other 'healthy' behaviours are often performed without conscious recognition of their contribution to health. Returning to McQueen's 'holy four' again, exercise provides a prime example. Blaxter (1990) suggests that, for the teenager, playing football is done for the pleasure of taking part, of simply doing it, rather than for its beneficial effects on cardiovascular efficiency or serum cholesterol level. Further, many behaviours regarded as undesirable by health professionals may represent important coping strategies for the individual.

From this review, we can see that lay models and theories of health and illness do exist and are by no means less important or valid than those of biomedicine; indeed, they are often more sophisticated. Although we have discussed lay beliefs as distinct from professional theory and opinion, it is important to recognize that professionals also hold their own 'lay' theories, which can be in conflict with their rational and scientific knowledge and understanding.

Lay Referral and Sectors of Health Care

It seems that it is not simply the presence of symptoms, but how the individual and those close to them *respond* to those symptoms that influences the decision to seek help or not. Helman (1990) believes that there are a number of questions that people typically ask themselves when they consider themselves ill. The answers they provide build up their theories of their illnesses that may be presented to their general practitioners. He suggests these questions are:

Reflection Points

Look at the following list of conditions, and jot down briefly what you know about them:

- chilblains
- piles
- dandruff
- spots
- flu
- greasy hair.

- Where does your knowledge of these conditions come from?
- How much does this knowledge differ from the medical establishment view?

(Exercise taken from Aggleton 1990)

1. *What has happened?* This includes organizing the symptoms into a pattern and giving them a name.
2. *Why has it happened?* This attempts to explain the possible cause(s).
3. *Why has it happened to me?* This tries to relate the illness to aspects of the person, such as behaviour, personality or temperament.
4. *Why now?* This concerns timing and speed of onset.
5. *What would happen to me if nothing were done about it?* This looks at the pros and cons of consulting, and includes possible outcomes and prognosis.
6. *What are its likely effects on other people* (family, friends, employers, etc.) *if nothing were done about it?* This addresses issues such as loss of income, or employment, and strain on relationships.
7. *What should I do about it – or to whom should I turn for further help?* Possible courses of action might include ignoring the symptoms, self-medication, consulting family and friends, *or* going to see the doctor.

These questions concur with Freidson's (1970) view that individuals have a lay referral system made up of a network of significant people, extending outside of the immediate family, and capable of influencing significantly their decision making. In other words, the individual seeks validation, be it implicit or explicit, from these people before choosing or not to see a doctor or other practitioner. If partners, friends and family are unwilling to define that individual as sick, they are then very unlikely to consult their doctor. Freidson further argues that an individual is more likely to consult their general practitioner when the members of their lay referral network share views and beliefs in line with that professional group. Working in the acute sector of the National Health Service (NHS), there is a tendency to assume that people with symptoms of one type or another will consult their general practitioner. But a growing number of people choose to consult outside of the 'official' health services. According to Fulder (1988), some 13% of the UK population consult a complementary practitioner each year, and there can be little doubt that these numbers are now much greater. In addition, Scambler (1991) cites evidence that approximately 35% of people attending a complementary practitioner had not consulted their

Box 3.2 Sectors of health care

- **Popular Sector** – 'where ill-health is first recognised and defined' (Helman 1990) – includes self-care, self-medication, talking to your granny or the vicar, going to bed, getting drunk or simply ignoring the symptoms. Hoarding of medication and exchanging medication amongst family and friends is very common in the UK.
- **Folk Sector** – ill-defined in this country. These methods of health care attempt to gain a holistic view of the individual. Options include spiritual and faith healers, palmists and clairvoyants as well as more legitimized practitioners such as homoeopaths.
- **Professional Sector** – includes the wide range of medical and paramedical options.

general practitioner with the problem in the first instance. This suggests that consultation with complementary practitioners is not simply a 'symptom' of dissatisfaction with traditional treatments, but also an indication of the increase in alternative health care options.

In most societies, people with emotional or physical difficulties do have a number of options open to them in terms of help. Generally, the more complex the society, the more of these options will be available, providing the individual can afford to pay (Helman 1990). This is termed *medical pluralism.* Although these options coexist, they are often based on entirely different theories and originate in different cultures. But as Helman points out, 'to the ill person, the origin of these treatments is less important than their efficacy in relieving suffering'.

One way of viewing the available health care options proposed by Kleinman (1980), is outlined in Box 3.2.

> The belief that medicine, grounded in the natural sciences, provides the only means of mediating between people and disease is being increasingly questioned, and there is a growing desire to explore alternative methods of health care which are both non-invasive and non-iatrogenic. (Rankin-Box 1989)

Predicting Behaviour

Some theorists have devised models that attempt to determine why people will or will not use preventative health services, or adopt a health-promoting lifestyle. One example is the Health Belief Model (Fig. 3.1). The model identifies the variables of susceptibility, severity of symptoms, benefits of change, and barriers to action *as perceived by the individual,* and further suggests that some form of 'trigger' initiates behaviour. The model has been criticized for merely presenting a number of variables rather than specifying the nature of the relationships between these variables. Although it was originally thought to predict those who would attend for immunization and smears, etc., it appears to explain only small variances in behaviour (Morgan *et al.* 1985). However, the model has been used extensively, and certainly may provide a useful mental checklist for nurses of the many factors which may influence decision making, but its ability to *predict* behaviour is inconsistent. Calnan's (1984) study of the take-up by women of early detection measures for breast cancer, found this model at best only weakly predictive of behaviour.

Kulbok (1985 cited by Pender 1987) describes a Resource Model of Preventative Health Behaviour, believing that people generally act in ways that maximize their 'stock in health'. In

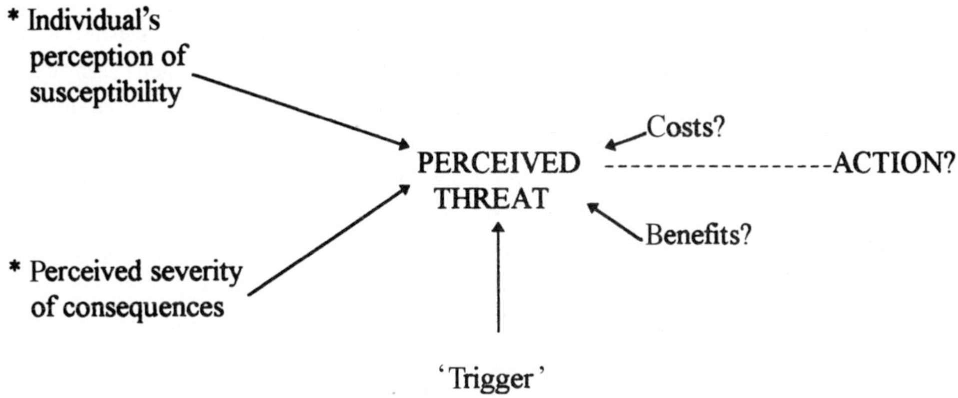

Figure 3.1 The Health Belief Model (Janz & Becker 1984)

short, the model suggests that the greater the social and health resources available to the individual, the more frequently they will engage in preventative behaviours. Health resources include the individual's perceived health status and energy, their concern or value placed on health and feelings about taking care of health, and participation in social groups. Kulbok also perceives the number of friends and relatives an individual has as a health resource (which concurs with Blaxter's (1990) view that it is *perceived* support rather than *actual* support that is most important in health protection and promotion), and goes on to define social resources as education and income.

According to Gillis (1993), the most frequently studied determinant of a health-promoting lifestyle is the individual's perceived control over their health. There are three aspects to the theory:

1. control by self (known as internal locus of control)
2. control by powerful others
3. control by chance (nos. 2 and 3 constituting external locus of control).

Again, although extensively quoted, there is little evidence to substantiate this theory's reliability as a predictor of behaviour. In a review of 23 studies between 1983 and 1991, Gillis suggests that *self-efficacy* – perceived ability to achieve – is the strongest predictor of an individual's likelihood to adopt a health-promoting lifestyle. It would seem, as Dines (1994) suggests, that *knowledge* of these influences is more likely to help day surgery nurses and other health educators explain, rather than predict, individual behaviour.

> Current research suggests little support for any assumption that, if people are well informed about the consequences for health of particular forms of behaviour, they will develop the appropriate attitudes and act in a way calculated to promote their health. There is still less evidence that people's statements of belief, intention or attitude are strongly associated with such behaviour and can be used to predict it. (Pill 1991)

Patterns of Consultation

The presence of an illness iceberg raises the concern about possible unmet need (Scambler 1991). However, at the same time, general practitioners complain about the tendency of people to consult for what they define as 'trivial' problems, which in turn has led to research into patterns of consultation. Repeated studies over the past 10 years, consistently demonstrate that women in the 17–44 age group go to the doctor twice as often as men (Verbrugge 1985). Although much of this excess may be explained by their need to attend for reproduction-related problems, when figures are controlled for all sex-specific conditions, there is still a female excess in consultation of approximately 30% (Verbrugge 1985). She further identifies more prescription of drugs to women in comparison to men, this being particularly noticeable in the 19–34 years age group.

Armstrong (1989) highlights the difficulty in separating the actual symptoms of a condition from their perception by the sufferer and their tolerance. Men are socialized very differently from women, and are usually expected to have what Helman (1990) describes as 'an unemotional language of distress' (see later in this chapter), to be stoical and uncomplaining. Nurses, too, are socialized to *expect* different responses to pain and anxiety, for example in the men and women in their care. Male and female nurses will, in turn, react differently to these responses. It is vital that these stereotyped gender expectations are challenged, and for nurses to encourage free expression of symptoms by all patients.

As pointed out earlier, men are known to under-report symptoms when compared to women (Clarke 1983); this may reflect their disinclination to admit to illness, as if it might be perceived as weakness. Women, on the other hand, as a result of complex socializing influences are more likely to define problems as illness and report them as such. The same socialization patterns help to familiarize women with health matters. They are reinforced not only by media images of a 'healthy' body and lifestyle, but also by the redefinition of normal physiological reproductive functions through the process of medicalization.

Medicalization is described as 'the way in which the jurisdiction of modern medicine has expanded in recent years and now encompasses many problems that formerly were not defined as medical entities' (Gabe & Calnan 1989). These authors further contend that, as such, the process constitutes an effective and powerful vehicle of social control that serves the interest of medicine with its increasing focus on disease rather than illness. Helman (1990) adds that the process of medicalization has been assisted by the undoubtedly successful and high-profile advances in medical technology, which serve to reinforce people's dependence on the medical profession for the solutions to their problems.

For women, the medicalization of their reproductive functions has had both beneficial and unwanted effects. The availability of symptom relief has been greatly welcomed, as women suffering from dysmenorrhoea, menorrhagia and premenstrual syndrome (PMS) will testify. However, whilst not denying the real distress suffered by many women, PMS provides a lucid example of how a biological event has come to be redefined as a pathological one. Defined as 'the commonest endocrine disorder' (Dalton, cited by Helman 1990), PMS has been attributed to a number of hormonal imbalances, for example progesterone, steroids and prolactin (Webb 1985). In defining these disturbances of mood as hormone-deficiency linked, medicine reinforces the stereotype of female supposed irrationality and anger as biologically based and therefore fixed. It also denies women the right to free expression of these feelings for their own sake.

Nevertheless, the predominance of the medical model largely results in other perspectives being marginalized or ignored (Pill 1991), whilst blaming the individual for feckless and irresponsible behaviour, and imposing professionally-held views remain common practice. As we will see, such approaches can have negative effects both on doctor–patient relationships, nurse–patient relationships and patient compliance with advice and treatment.

Negotiating the Consultation

> Far from the outcome of the consultation being determined only by the problem that the patient brings and by the diagnosis of the doctor, the outcome is a result of mutual interaction. (Stimson & Webb 1975)

Morgan (1991) estimates that in excess of half a million meetings between general practitioners and patients take place every working day. The average consultation is less than 10 min, and in that time both doctor and patient need to negotiate their way through a potential mire of questions, answers, misunderstandings, obscure terminology, frustrations, impatience and embarrassment before any diagnosis or treatment options are even discussed. Even then, not all symptoms or the patient's *real* problem will necessarily have been disclosed.

Much therefore depends on general practitioners first creating the right environment for patients to present their problems, and second, having the necessary communication skills to facilitate a sensitive discussion. Helman draws our attention to what he calls the 'languages of distress'; that is, the ways in which we communicate our suffering to others, including doctors. They may be verbal or non-verbal, and clearly differ between and within socio-cultural and gender groups. Helman suggests that doctors who are unable to decipher these 'codes' may be in danger of misinterpreting the symptoms and making the wrong diagnosis, a situation more likely if the patient and doctor are from different socio-cultural or gender groups.

For example, evidence suggests that the predominantly male medical profession is more likely to diagnose neurotic conditions in women than in men (Clarke 1983, Turner 1987, Miles 1988). Turner describes a 'mutually reinforcing' situation, where women report more symptoms to doctors who have been trained to expect them to do just that. Miles (1988) recognizes the comparative ease of seeing a general practitioner as opposed to a social worker or family counsellor. It could therefore be assumed that if women are taking social problems to the doctor because access to other help is problematic, and in turn the doctor interprets the problem in psychological terms and prescribes psychotropic drugs, both the female excess of consultation and use of tranquillizers can be readily explained. So, it is difficult to assess whether greater self-reports of symptoms by women are representative of a greater health need or more a feature of illness behaviour and a different language of distress.

Further evidence of communication difficulties during consultation is gained from a study of some 300 patients in general practice undertaken by Tuckett and colleagues in 1985. Their findings indicate that information given during a consultation is frequently forgotten or misunderstood. Interestingly, these authors also revealed a statistically significant relationship between the doctor's lack of interest in the patient's point of view as perceived by the patient, and subsequent poor compliance with treatment. This evaluation of their general practitioner's interest generally occurs *after* the consultation. Stimson and Webb (1975) argue that this and other notable processes, that is, making sense of what has happened and reappraisal of original theories of symptoms also occur *after* the patient has left the surgery.

Although these research studies have been conducted with patients and doctors, some parallels can be drawn between this phenomenon and patients' attendance at a nurse-run pre-assessment clinic. It is indeed possible that if patients perceive nurses to be more interested in *giving* standard information than listening to their concerns, that co-operation with pre-operative preparation may be lessened.

So the lay referral network still has an important role to play in whether or not the patient complies with prescribed treatment, therefore highlighting the paradoxical nature of general practice. 'In the consultation, the doctor makes the treatment decisions: after the consultation, decision making lies with the patient' (Stimson & Webb 1975).

Pill (1991) believes that many clinicians are now becoming more aware that many communication difficulties between themselves and their patients during consultation often arise from misunderstandings of what to them, is very simple terminology. Morgan (1991) adds that patients' descriptions are often just as likely to be misunderstood by the doctor. However, despite this growing awareness, evidence from patient satisfaction studies suggests that many general practitioners still rely on the traditional and paternalistic 'doctor knows best' approach. More active attempts on their behalf to elicit their patients' beliefs and understandings, and help them make sense of often complex information and treatment options, may well achieve greater compliance and improved outcomes. Adopting a similar approach would likewise prove beneficial for nurses in day surgery in their attempts to improve patient compliance with both pre- and postoperative advice and instructions.

Patients' Expectations

Sutherland (1991) in an account of day surgery practice emphasizes the importance of setting up systems and protocols to provide a first-class service. In order to provide such a service, staff need to be 'flexible, innovative and technically proficient'. She also mentions how patients often have unrealistic and erroneous expectations of day surgery. There is little doubt that these experiences are shared by day surgery nurses across the country, and certainly it is the case within our own unit. But none the less, they are simply *views*; they do not represent the findings of any empirical study. Not that this renders the observation invalid, but it is important to recognize both the limitations and the potential hazards associated with anecdotal accounts of patient behaviour. The patients appear to be mocked, albeit gently, for their dismay at having such unrealistic expectations corrected.

The more important and somewhat arrogant aspect of this account is the implicit suggestion that the *patients really should have known better*. But why should they? Why do we presume that an individual, often with no prior experience of being in hospital, should acquire this knowledge before attending for pre-assessment? In fact, Sutherland (1991), whilst chiding patients for not knowing better, in the next paragraph explicitly recognizes that many of the patients attending her unit are having their first surgical 'encounter'! Given our understanding of lay logic and interpretation of symptoms and treatment options, it does appear quite logical to assume that having surgery as a day case equates with minimal disruption to normal life and activity. It does appear that despite greater awareness amongst nurses of individual differences, patients are still classified into one of two stereotyped groups, both of which are based on the false assumption that health and health care are priorities in everyone's lives:

- those who have some knowledge and understanding, but sometimes ask difficult questions and have overly high expectations (i.e. they know too much for their own good) and,

- those who apparently know little, are not interested in finding out more, and have few expectations (i.e. they're not very bright and wouldn't understand the information anyway).

Patients therefore are open to criticism, for both asking and not asking, questions. In a study of decision-making in a day unit, Avis (1992) argues that there is generally too much information *giving* at the expense of information *sharing*, but also makes the important point that the patients largely *expected the interactions to be that way*. Most of the information that the patients in this study had procured about their condition (inguinal hernia) and their forthcoming operation, they had obtained from friends and relatives with experience of the same problem (the lay referral network). They then adopted a more 'traditional' and passive patient role during consultation with the surgeon, because they believed that they would be *told* what they needed to know.

Although a small and qualitative study, its findings are important and in the light of this knowledge, perhaps it is not so surprising that differences both in patients' expectations and understanding are demonstrated. Similarly, being told by a doctor or nurse that the forthcoming operation is only a *minor* one, clearly indicates another area where the expectations associated with that description do not match the reality of often considerable postoperative discomfort. Vague and ambiguous terms like 'minor' and 'major' should be avoided in discussions with patients about their conditions and surgery.

Dutton (1994) suggests that as patients are consumers, their involvement in their care is vital. But do patients consider themselves as consumers of health care? Avis's study suggests that far from seeing themselves as partners in the process, patients 'expect to be told what to do and would rather hand over the responsibility for decision making to the professionals'. He argues that although day surgery rates highly in terms of patient satisfaction, it does not seem to offer choice and participation, describing more a climate in which professionals give, rather than share information. Similar concerns about patients being coerced into participation are discussed by Waterworth and Luker (1990) and Biley (1992). Of further interest is the patient's tendency to regard any postoperative complication as an indication of their poor decision to have surgery on a day basis (Avis 1992). In selecting the day or inpatient option for surgery however, all the patients in this study deferred to the knowledge and status of the professionals. Avis rightly warns that strategies to increase patient involvement in decision-making may result in an increased likelihood of patients blaming themselves when things go wrong.

Summary

Research into health beliefs has provided substantial evidence of the existence of distinct and sophisticated lay models, although little indication has emerged that knowledge of such beliefs can help nurses predict behaviour. However, knowledge and acceptance of these alternative views reinforces the unique individuality of all people requiring health care and may help nurses in the area of day surgery understand and explain the different ways in which patients respond to illness and surgery. More notably, this chapter has reminded us of the need to put health and illness in perspective; to avoid what Dines (1994) refers to as 'healthism' and recognize the importance of other values and goals in people's lives.

Key points

- Differences in opinion do exist between different professional groups (e.g. doctors and nurses) and between professional groups and the public.
- Lay beliefs of health and illness are no less important or valid than those of the professionals; in fact they are often more sophisticated.
- Lay beliefs differ between and within societies, are subject to change over generations, and are therefore culturally determined, and shaped by socialization processes.
- Individuals largely fail to recognize their own contribution to their being ill, but they do feel responsible for not looking after their health.
- Professionals also hold 'lay' beliefs about causes of disease and illness; beliefs often at odds with their own professional knowledge and understanding.
- Illness behaviour and patterns of consultation differ between gender and age groups, are influenced by available lay referral networks and are reinforced by both social and biomedical stereotypes.
- Patient compliance is clearly influenced by attitudes and communication skills of clinicians *and* nurses.
- Policies to increase patient involvement in decision-making do not necessarily match patient expectations.
- Eliciting health beliefs of patients is an essential prerequisite to effective health education.
- All health professionals need to avoid a 'healthist' approach, and accept the different priorities in the lives of others.

Recommended Reading

Blaxter, M. (1990) **Health and Lifestyles**. London: Tavistock/Routledge

Interesting and challenging account of health in the 1980s

Helman, C. (1990) **Culture, Health and Illness** (Second Edition). Oxford: Butterworth–Heinemann

A comprehensive and quite fascinating insight into the cultural factors influencing our health

Naidoo, J. and Wills, J. (1994) **Health Promotion: Foundations for practice**. London: Baillière Tindall

The definitive text on health and health promotion

References

Aggleton, P. (1990) **Health**. London: Routledge.

Armstrong, D. (1989) **An Outline of Sociology as Applied to Medicine** (Third Edition). London: Wright.

Avis, M. (1992) **Silent partners – patients' views about choice and decision making in a day unit.** *British Journal of Theatre Nursing* **2**(7): 8–11.

Backett, K. (1990) **Image and reality. Health enhancing behaviours in middle class families.** *Health Education Journal* **49**(2): 61–63.

Backett, K. (1991) **Talking to young children about health: methods and findings.** *Health Education Journal* **50**(1): 34–38.

Biley, F. (1992) **In defence of the passive patient.** *Nursing Times* **88**(21): 58.

Blaxter, M. and Paterson L. (1982) **Mothers and daughters: A three generation study of health attitudes and behaviour**. London: Heinemann.

Blaxter, M. (1990) **Health and Lifestyles**. London: Tavistock/Routledge.

Calnan, M. (1984) **The Health Belief Model and participation in programmes for the early detection of breast cancer: a comparative analysis.** *Social Science & Medicine* **19**: 823–830.

Calnan, M. (1987) **Health and Illness: The lay perspective**. London: Tavistock.

Clarke, J. (1983) **Sexism, feminism and medicalism: a decade of literature on gender and illness.** *Sociology of Health and Illness* **5**(1): 61–82.

Cornwell, J. (1984) **Hard Earned Lives: Accounts of health and illness from East London**. London: Tavistock.

Davies, B. M. (1991) **Community Health & Social Services** (Fifth Edition). London: Edward Arnold.

Dines, A. (1994) **A review of lay health beliefs research: insights for nursing practice in health promotion.** *Journal of Clinical Nursing* **3**: 329–338.

Dutton, K. E. A. (1994) **Patient education in a day surgery unit.** *Journal of One-Day Surgery* **Spring**: 22–24.

Elkind, A., Haran, D., Eardley, A., Spencer, B. and Smith, A. (1989) **Computer managed call and recall for cervical screening: a topology of reasons for non-attendance.** *Community Medicine* **11**(2): 157–162.

Freidson, E. (1970) **The Profession of Medicine**. New York: Dodd-Mead.

Fulder, S. (1988) **The Handbook of Complementary Medicine**. London: Coronet.

Gabe, J. and Calnan, M. (1989) **The limits of medicine: women's perception of medical technology.** *Social Science & Medicine* **28**(3): 223–231.

Gillis, A. J. (1993) **Determinants of a health-promoting lifestyle: an integrative review.** *Journal of Advanced Nursing* **18**: 345–353.

Hannay, D. R. (1988) **Lecture Notes on Medical Sociology**. Oxford: Blackwell Scientific.

Helman, C. (1990) **Culture, Health and Illness** (Second Edition). Oxford: Butterworth–Heinemann.

Herzlich, C. (1973) **Health and Illness: A social psychological analysis**. London: Academic Press.

Jacobson, B., Smith, A. and Whitehead, M. (1991) **The Nation's Health: A Strategy for the 1990s** (Second Edition). London: Kings Fund.

Janz, N. K. and Becker, M. H. (1984) **The Health Belief Model: a decade later.** *Health Education Quarterly* **11**: 1–47.

Kleinman, A. (1980) **Patients and Healers in the Context of Culture**. Berkeley: University of California Press.

Martin, J. and Main, P. J. (1992) **Cervical screening: default and compliance.** *Health Visitor* **65**(4): 123–124.

Mechanic, D. (1968) **Medical Sociology**. New York: Free Press.

Miles, A. (1988) **Women and Mental Illness**. Brighton: Wheatsheaf Books.

Morgan, M. (1991) **The doctor–patient relationship.** In Scambler G. (Ed) *Sociology as Applied to Medicine* (Third Edition). London: Baillière Tindall.

Morgan, M., Calnan, M. and Manning, N. (1985) **Sociological Approaches to Health and Medicine**. London: Routledge.

Naidoo, J. and Wills, J. (1994) **Health Promotion: Foundations for practice**. London: Baillière Tindall.

Nathanson, C. (1977) **Sex, illness and medical care: a review of data, theory and method.** *Social Science & Medicine* **11**: 13–25.

Orem, D. E. (1985) **Nursing: Concepts of practice** (Third Edition). New York: McGraw-Hill.

Pender, N. (1987) **Health Promotion in Nursing Practice** (Second Edition). Norwalk, CT: Appleton & Lange.

Pill, R. (1991) **Issues in lifestyles and health: lay meanings of health and health behaviour.** In Badura, B. & Kickbusch, I. (Eds) *Health Promotion Research: Towards a new social epidemiology.* WHO Regional Publications.

Pill, R. and Stott, N. (1982) **Concepts of illness causation and responsibility: some preliminary data from a sample of working class mothers.** *Social Science & Medicine* **16**: 43–52.

Pill, R. and Stott, N. (1985) **Choice or chance: further evidence on ideas of illness and responsibility for health.** *Social Science & Medicine* **20**: 981–991.

Rankin-Box, D. F. (Ed) (1989) **Complementary Health Therapies: A guide for nurses and the caring professions**. London: Croom Helm.

Royal College of Surgeons for England (1985) **Guidelines for day surgery**. London: HMSO.

Royal College of Surgeons for England (1992) **Report of the working party on guidelines for day case surgery** (Revised Edition). London: RCoS.

Scambler, G. and Scambler, A. (1984) **The illness iceberg and aspects of consulting behaviour.** In Fitzpatrick R. *et al. The Experience of Illness.* London: Tavistock.

Scambler, G. (Ed) (1991) **Sociology as Applied to Medicine** (Third Edition). London: Baillière Tindall.

Stimson, G. and Webb, B. (1975) **Going to See the Doctor**. London: Routledge & Kegan Paul.

Sutherland, E. (1991) **All in a day's work.** *Nursing Times* **87**(11): 26–30.

Tuckett, D., Boulton, M., Olson, C. and Williams, A. (1985) **Meetings between experts: An approach to sharing ideas in medical consultations**. London: Tavistock.

Turner, B. S. (1987) **Medical Power & Social Knowledge**. London: Sage.

Verbrugge, L. (1985) **Gender and health: an update on hypotheses and evidence.** *Journal of Health & Social Behaviour* **26**: 156–182.

Waterworth, A. and Luker, K. (1990) **Reluctant collaborators: do patients want to be involved in decisions regarding care?** *Journal of Advanced Nursing* **15**: 971–976.

Webb, C. (1985) **Sexuality, Nursing and Health**. Chichester: John Wiley.

Whitehead, M. (1988) **The Health Divide: Inequalities in Health**. London: Penguin.

Williams, R. (1983) **Concepts of health: an analysis of lay logic.** *Sociology* **17**: 185–205.

Chapter 4 Communication needs

Terry Wilson

Overview

The communication needs of patients are an area of concern across the whole National Health Service (NHS). We argue here that they remain of central concern within the day surgery setting and that nurses need to guard against believing that technical and technological wizardry, as well as rapid turnover of patients, militate against effective use of the so called 'soft' skills of nursing – listening, responding and providing accurate information.

A simple model or framework for communication is provided which, we hope, will encourage the reader to consider communication from the perspective of the consumer, that is, 'what does this patient want and need from me?' rather than from the perspective of the organization, that is, 'what do we want to offer given the time we've got'. Whilst we do not want to take a foolishly unrealistic stance we would like to reopen the debate about what is possible in nurse–patient communication in a relatively short interaction.

Chapter Focus

- Evidence of nurses' existing communication skills
- Five Levels of Helping (Wilson 1996) and their application in day surgery
- Information giving
- Maximizing skills and time

Introduction

Sadly, the literature on nurse–patient communication has repeatedly indicated that nurses:

- label and stereotype patients (Stockwell 1972)
- defend themselves from getting involved with patients (Menzies 1960, Macleod-Clark 1984, Wright 1991) and
- engage in short interactions of around 3 min (Faulkner 1981, Bond 1983).

Studies in specific areas, for example intensive care (Ashworth 1980), surgical wards (Macleod-Clark 1981), in relation to pain relief (Hayward 1975) and even with student nurses (Gott 1984), have all highlighted deficiencies in both quantity and quality. The fact that many of these studies are more than 10 years old might tempt us to believe that they are outdated and inaccurate and that the world has moved on since then. This is apparently not the case, even if we allow for the fact that traditional Registered General Nurse (RGN) programmes allowed little room for communication skills and that Project 2000 courses have yet to produce sufficient practitioners to effect a culture shift. This incidentally assumes they are better communicators, which in itself may be questionable.

Rather than make assumptions about whether nurses in day surgery communicate better or worse, it seems more useful to suggest that all patients are individual and their needs are unique and idiosyncratic. They require time, they require information and they want to be listened to (rather than be blocked or dismissed). There is no evidence to suggest that the needs of day surgery patients are any different. Responding to these needs demands that nurses possess the skills, the desire and the motivation to get involved with patients, even though they are only there for a short period of time. In addition, nurses need the ability to cope with the emotional demands patient involvement brings, as well as working in an environment where this is valued and where workload is such that it is seen as feasible.

In day surgery, knowing how best to respond, or identifying what the needs of patients are can be problematic. We have found the following framework useful in ensuring that the level of help given is what patients want and not simply what nurses habitually give. When a large number of patients are perceived by nurses as requiring the 'same' information, it is very likely that the same approach will be adopted. No matter how well intentioned this help might be, it is only useful in as much as it meets patients' perceived needs. This certainly accords with Rogers (1961) writings and follows a principle of being non-directive or client centred, but it will be seen that there are points at which we diverge from that principle.

Levels of Helping

The following levels of helping should clarify the purposes of different approaches and assist the nurse in selecting the approach most suited to each unique situation.

The five levels of help were arrived at in response to the question 'What do patients want and need from nurses?'. Answers to this seem to include the need or desire for practical help, information, a listening ear, advice or for counselling. These are sometimes very clear and mutually exclusive, some patients will just want 'to get it fixed' (Avis 1992) and view offers of emotional support and information as an unwelcome intrusion.

However, as highlighted in Chapter 3, Helman (1990) indicates that there are seven questions which are often around for patients. At first glance questions such as:

- What has happened?
- What would happen if nothing were done about it?
- What should I do about it?

look like requests for information yet each is also a part of what he describes as the search for the meaning of the experience. Tschudin (1995) asks 'What is the meaning of it?' as the third of her

Box 4.1 Levels of Helping (Wilson 1996)

1. Practical help	**Doing**
2. Giving information	**Informing**
3. Allowing the patient to ventilate feelings	**Listening**
4. Enabling the patient to identify the problem	**Challenging**
5. Helping the patient to manage the problem	**Counselling**

four questions in her model of counselling and it becomes apparent that in asking questions about meaning patients may want

- information – Level 2
- to be listened to, as they express their concern or confusion – Level 3
- help in sorting out the confusion – Level 5
- all of these in different doses.

Decisions about which level to respond at are often made on the basis of the whole story, non-verbal cues and other indicators. However, there are occasions when it is difficult to work out what patients really want, or we have a hunch that patients are saying one thing but actually asking another. In these circumstances, asking directly what sort of help patients want seems to be the most fruitful and respectful approach; it ensures that the choice remains with patients. It also lessens the doubt and the internal dialogue of nurses (how often have you found yourself listening to a patient, trying to take in what they are saying, preparing your next reply, and wondering whether you are doing it right or missing something important?) and, perhaps most importantly, it signals to patients that they have choices. In other words it is clear statement that patients have *permission* to take some control over the choice of content, nurses are prepared to *share* the process and the aim is that it is a *partnership*.

1. Practical Help

The sorts of practical help patients may seek are, of course, manifold, and outside the scope of this particular chapter. However, there is an issue of appropriateness and timing. Too much help can contribute to a level of dependency and learned helplessness whereas too little help may, at worst, be construed as neglect and malpractice, and at best, as insensitivity.

The bottom line, in considering which level of help might apply in a given situation is provided in the answer to the following two questions:

- What does the patient want and need at this moment?
- What am I paid to provide (i.e. what is my contract with this individual)?

In many nursing situations including day surgery, patients require physical care and nurses traditionally respond to these needs. Consequently, level one interventions come most easily or most naturally to nurses. But these 'natural' skills have taken years of learning, shaping and developing to become part of the skilled practitioner's repertoire. Consequently, they are integrated and habitual in the way that an advanced driver can 'mirror, signal and manoeuvre' without actually having to think about it.

Far less time is devoted, in the total nursing curriculum, to learning how best to communicate with patients. This often seems to be left to chance and the assumption that 'communicating is easy, we do it all the time'. We would argue that effective communication involves a range of skills which need to be applied at the right time to produce maximum effect. These skills can be learnt, mislearnt and unlearnt but, ultimately, when used well will seem 'natural' and integrated.

On inpatient wards nurses will often have time to build up rapport, develop the relationship and respond to patients' needs. There is some scope for getting it wrong, because the opportunity is there for patients to ask further questions or for nurses to volunteer further information.

However, in day surgery there is more pressure to get it right first time. Therefore, the need for adequate preparation and training of nurses in communication skills is increased, as is the requirement for individual practitioners to reflect upon their performance and seek support and supervision.

2. Giving Information

Classic studies by Boore (1978) and Hayward (1975) indicate that pre-operative information-giving reduces pain and discomfort as well as lessening anxiety. The Audit Commission (1991) questionnaire on patient experience suggests an improvement in information-giving which is in contrast to the findings of Bowling (1992). Her examination of the literature on patient satisfaction in day surgery found generally uncritical responses about the care given. She highlights a study in North Bedfordshire which indicated that 66% patients had received no instructions on how to cope with the after effect of their treatment and a number complained about transport arrangements. These are useful reminders to us that information-giving should not stop at an explanation of the procedure but must include practical arrangements and especially follow-up care.

Pre-admission assessment has been emphasized in recent literature (Murphy 1994) but it is worth noting that such assessment, especially when it is known as *pre-screening,* is often more concerned with identifying patients' *suitability* for surgery. On the other hand, a pre-operative assessment that incorporates *information-giving* about the procedure, facilities and aftercare not only enhances the quality of the assessment but goes further towards meeting patient need. (For more in-depth information about pre-admission assessment please refer to Chapter 5.) Individual nurses claim they can assess patients' suitability, give information, provide reassurance and emotional support, and counsel the patient during these brief meetings! Perhaps the purpose of the assessment needs to be more clear and focused and unrealistic expectations avoided, since it does seem that pre-admission assessment varies enormously between units. They are also sometimes omitted due to pressure of work, staff shortages and perhaps a sense that they are not essential (Johnson 1990).

Conversely, when talking with a group of trained nurses about the skills required in giving information and the subtleties of matching the approach to patient need we found that in some instances, pre-admission assessment was taking place 12 months in advance of the actual admission. When we questioned the benefit of this assessment, the response was that it does not matter whether patients retain any of the information, what is important is that it has been done and can be ticked off the list of tasks. In this instance, pre-admission assessment was yet another routine task to complete and any audit which solely measures behaviours will see this as a job well done.

Menzies (1960) highlighted the many ways in which nurses protect themselves from getting close to patients, among which were stereotyping and task orientation. The nursing process, primary nursing, and the increase in communication skills within the nursing curriculum were supposed to lead to greater holism and individual approaches to patient care. However, Wright (1991) points out that nurses have developed a whole new series of mechanisms to avoid getting too close to patients, among which he identifies reliance on over-documentation, complaints about staffing levels and workloads, and a need to adhere to policies and procedures. These are certainly cries frequently to be heard on a day unit. Certainly, the above anecdote indicates that documentation and following procedures were taking place at the expense of any meaningful interaction.

Whilst the nursing literature (Alcock 1986, Hathaway 1986, Swindale 1989) is replete with evidence that information giving is a good thing, it is interesting to note that there is little information in the literature on *how* to give information. The necessity for information is made abundantly clear, but:

- what information to give
- under what circumstances
- by whom
- and in what form or volume

is rarely discussed in either nursing or communication texts. Brammer (1993) goes so far as to say that the skill 'is so commonplace that it needs little elaboration'. Burnard and Morrison (1989) in a study of nurses' perceptions of their interpersonal skills, found that nurses rated themselves highly with respect to providing support, giving information and telling patients what to do, and less highly at confronting patients, facilitating emotions and encouraging patients to talk.

However, it seems that the first question to ask is 'should I give this information at all?'. At one level this can be seen as an ethical or professional dilemma – should patients be told their diagnosis up front, only when the question is asked, piecemeal or only when it is absolutely confirmed? This is the dilemma faced by medical staff on a regular basis following investigations and the ways of dealing with this vary enormously.

The ways in which this is handled may lead to problems for nurses. How do we deal with patients who want to know what doctors mean when they say it was a 'wart' or 'not very nasty'? Do we clarify for these patients, avoid them, refer them to the doctor? Or do we become anxious, angry and annoyed with a system that allows medical staff to put us in that awkward situation (forgetting for the moment that they, too, are human and have to find a way of dealing with the enormity of the situation)?

It is interesting to note that approaches to breaking bad news and giving a diagnosis are complicated by a tension between 'what I would like if it were me' and a worry about patients' responses – they may shout, or they may become seriously distressed – 'Will I be able to cope?'.

Reflection Points

- Recall (if you have been in this position) the last time you were very ill, but had not received a diagnosis or confirmation of what was wrong (you may even have been awaiting the results of investigations).
- What were your worst thoughts and fears, especially in the quiet hours of the night when you had time to let your fantasies run away with you?
- You may already have seen a terminal illness, your funeral, the effects of your demise on loved ones and still had time to tell yourself off for being silly.

However, it could be argued that failure to be honest and upfront with information is ultimately more damaging to patients who are already likely to be catastrophizing and creating a worst-case scenario in their head. They are also likely to be struggling with the possibility that they are being 'silly', overreacting and that it cannot be that bad or the nurses and doctors would have told them.

In other words, human nature being what it is, patients will most probably have guessed or anticipated the worst and stoically arrived bracing themselves for that information, particularly if a friend has been for a bronchoscopy or they have read about it or talked to people. Lack of honesty is akin to being overprotective, in the way that we often are with our children who may resent not having gone to Grandma's funeral and feel betrayed in some way. Loss of trust is the possible consequence, and repair of that can be difficult. Our point here is that the nurses need to ask themselves whether their desire to withhold information is really because patients will not be able to deal with it, based on a sound assessment of individual patients, or whether it is about protecting themselves and putting their own needs for comfort ahead of patients' needs for information.

The other side to deciding whether to give information is more practical. The question to ask is whether patients are really requesting information or whether they are really looking for an opportunity to talk or express fears. 'How often should I take the tablets for?' or 'How long should the dressing stay on?' would seem like reasonable requests for factual information. However, questions such as 'The doctor says I should give up smoking, what do you think?' or 'I'm really worried about what is going to happen' may be requests for information which will be helpful and reassuring or they may be prompts from patients that this is an issue they would like to talk about more fully.

Making the decision about whether to give information, which might constitute premature reassurance and close down the conversation, or to explore what patients are really asking might, at first glance, seem quite difficult. Certainly, practical considerations such as time, workload, and absence or presence of privacy may play a part in this but it would seem reasonable to ask; 'I'm not sure what you're asking, whether you want a direct answer or you want to talk to me about this?'.

In other words, decisions about which route to take do not always have to rest with the nurse. The skill of clarifying, or checking uncertainty (Tschudin 1995) can be used to determine the direction of the conversation and remain truly patient centred.

If it is obvious that information is required then the next issue is

- how much?
- who should deliver it?
- and how?

Certain principles would seem to apply and at its simplest level, the 'News at Ten' approach – tell them what you are going to say, say it, and then tell them what you have said – is most useful. Other issues are also critical:

Step One

- Get the environment right – is it private enough?
- Try to minimize external distractions. A patient will find it difficult to listen if their 3 year old is climbing all over them.

- check on patients' readiness for the information – they may be distracted by the need to get out to pick up a child from school.

In some ways these distractions may be minimized by arranging pre-admission assessment at a time more suitable for individual patients which might not be on the day of consultation (see Chapter 5). In more detail, we would argue that it is vital to note and respond to patients' non-verbal messages throughout the whole process of information-giving or patient teaching. Egan (1994) writes about the concept of *non-verbal leakage*, suggesting that patients may censor the verbal message but find it difficult to censor the non-verbal one. Thus, patients often feel obliged or indebted to the 'nice and busy' nurse who is explaining something as well as suffering from the human frailty of not wishing to appear foolish and therefore may claim to have understood an explanation whilst still looking puzzled or confused. In this instance, the observant nurse will respond to the non-verbal message and give patients the opportunity to check out what they do not understand.

If this is an overriding principle to bear in mind throughout the whole process then we should also:

Step Two

Check out what patients already know and what they would like to know, have expanded or clarified. This would seem to us to be vitally important because:

- It is a patient-centred starting point and will allow a reasonable assessment of where to start and what to include, rather than being presumptive.
- Patients will have seen other health professionals and may either have been given different information, or more probably, interpreted and remembered the information in different ways, bearing in mind our earlier observations (Chapter 3) about lay beliefs of health and illness.

Step Three

The next step would be to *plan* what to explain, in what sequence, and using what medium. This may seem self-evident but how many of us allow ourselves the luxury, consistently, to plan what we are going to say and take a proactive rather than merely reactive approach to information giving? Too much planning may, of course be unhelpful; it is impossible to predict how the session will go if we are going to be flexible and responsive to patients' needs.

However, consideration should be given to:

- what points need to be made and emphasized
- ensuring that information given is accurate
- using language that is jargon-free yet precise and clear, as well as appropriate to the age, culture and gender of patients
- what points need to be emphasized and re-emphasized with diagrams, descriptions, written information or demonstrations.

Perhaps a key point is to recap and summarize information at regular points, with the clear invitation for patients to ask about parts they may have misunderstood. A useful question here is 'who should recap?'. It could be argued that the nurse should do it to ensure that they have given the right information but it might be more useful if the patients themselves do it, since this will give a clear indication of what has been recalled and what has been subject to a different interpretation or emphasis.

Step Four

Give the information, as indicated above and

Step Five

Check for understanding, as indicated above.

Reflection Points

- Recall an occasion when you have recently explained a procedure to a patient.
- What do you believe you did well?
- What might you have improved upon, or done differently?
- Now consider giving that same information to another patient.
- How might it change if the patient is older, younger, of a different gender, from a different culture?

You might wish to consider whether you would become more, or less, detailed; whether you would change your examples or analogies; whether you would provide more written information or other visual aids; and on what you would base those decisions.

We would like here to make a clear distinction between *information*-giving and *advice*-giving. The former would seem to be about imparting knowledge, information, even choices or options without applying any value to it, for example 'Your options might be to have chemotherapy, have radiotherapy with chemotherapy or to choose to do neither', while the latter is more about offering an opinion based upon your own personal or professional knowledge.

In most cases we would suggest that advice-giving is inadvisable and generally unhelpful, especially if this is based on the helper's personal view of how they would deal with a situation. However, there is a case for saying that health professionals have a discrete body of knowledge and a wealth of experience about disease processes, treatment and prognosis and that failure to share that with patients is actually denying them access to valuable information which may be helpful.

However, we would continue to argue that helping patients to identify the options and come up with their own choice is the most empowering approach and we would call this information-giving. Thereafter, there may be situations where it is helpful to give information about what choices other patients have made in these circumstances, while still leaving the final choice to the individual. It is very natural that patients will ask directly for advice but the smart nurse will generally enable patients to explore the situation by starting with information-giving and then moving to ventilation of feelings and a problem-solving approach. In other words, the whole process is about sharing information and engaging in a *dialogue* rather than a monologue.

3. Allowing Patients to Ventilate Feelings

Surprisingly, this is often very difficult for nurses to do. Merely listening can seem a very passive and unproductive activity, even more so for men who like to come up with *solutions* to problems rather than actually *listen* to the problem. We have also noticed that participants on counselling courses are often so keen to get into problem-solving that they do so before they have actually accurately identified the problem; this also happens with friends who offer well-intentioned advice before they have fully appreciated the nature of the problem.

Non-defensive listening can be especially difficult, although necessary, if patients are complaining about previous treatment, or 'the system'. It is tempting to defend these people, put forward alternatives or make it clear that you do not want to hear these opinions. However, non-defensive listening is vital and invaluable. Being listened to and understood can be a truly energizing and empowering experience. If nurses can do this with integrity and genuine concern for the viewpoint of patients then trust is enhanced, and it is possible that the conversation may well move from this level to needing information or help to problem-solve.

In other words, *listening is the first step* to each of the other levels of help. Failure to listen in the first instance will beget problems. Again, we would argue that the issue with regard to eliciting, listening to and responding to feelings is one of choice. We argued in the previous chapter that we are not advocating that nurses spend all their time getting details and feelings about the illness from noticing first symptoms, and accept the limitations of time. None the less, it is worth asking yourself whether you *generally* listen to the patients' expression of feelings, whether you *generally* respond by making reassuring noises or whether you *generally* steer away from these because it seems like uncomfortable territory.

In a wide range of communication skills' programmes with nurses from all sorts of settings, including day surgery and critical care, there is a consistent tendency to find nurses are very comfortable with asking questions and find paraphrasing content or reflecting feelings very difficult.

This is because, we would argue, these two skills are culturally abnormal. To the statement; 'I'm really worried about the anaesthetic and what's going to happen to me', nurses would appear

Learning Points

- **Reflection** – identifying the feelings expressed by the patient and putting these back to him/her. These feelings may be overtly or covertly expressed.
- **Paraphrase** – listening to what the patient is saying and putting the essential meaning (content) into other words.

The essential difference between the two skills is that reflection is about emphasizing feelings whereas paraphrazing is about content. There is no doubt that there are grey areas in distinguishing between the two, but it is important to note that both skills are used in an attempt to demonstrate understanding and not to steer or move the conversation into any new direction.

Reflection Points

- Practise by listening to a friend, or partner. Let them know that you are practising reflecting feelings. After a couple of minutes of listening see if you can accurately put back what this person has just said to you. Ask how accurate you were.
- If this goes well, repeat and keep up the practise. Discuss the impact of accurate reflection upon your partner.
- If it proves to be difficult we recommend you practise even more. The fact that it is difficult for you indicates it might be worthwhile for you to persevere.
- To get a real sense of the impact of reflecting think about a time when you felt truly listened to and understood. Identify what was going on then. What was the other person doing which was so useful?

more likely to ask; 'What are you worried for?' or to immediately explain that there is nothing to worry about; the anaesthetist is sober; everyone worries, its normal; you've got the best doctor we have; or 'trust me I'm a nurse'.

It seems less likely that the nurse would say; 'So you're both scared by the anaesthetic, and uncertain about the treatment' (*reflection* of feelings) or 'So you're unclear about what is going to happen' (*paraphrase* of content).

These responses alone, are geared to just letting patients know that you have heard their concerns accurately and serve as prompts to encourage patients to elaborate and say more about their concerns or the situation. Each is also a fundamental way of conveying empathy (Rogers 1961). There is clear behavioural evidence that the nurse has heard and restated what the patient is actually feeling or saying at that time which is patently not the case in the overused and frequently inaccurate 'I know just how you feel'.

Perhaps we need to make a point about questions here. In communication skills training it becomes apparent that some people overuse questions, and that the questions which they often overuse are closed and leading! There is a massive difference in the range of potential responses to 'How do you feel about your treatment?' (open question inviting a range of answers) and 'So, you don't feel worried about your treatment, do you?' (closed and leading question inviting the answer 'No').

We often hear people commencing questions with:

- do you feel ...
- do you think ...
- did you ....

all of which will start to lead the patient in the direction of the nurse. These sorts of questions may involve assumptions on the part of the questioner or may actually be a sloppy questioning habit from someone who is accurately picking up what the patient is thinking or feeling. To be asked, 'do you feel upset?' can lead to the answer 'haven't you been listening? I just said I was!' or 'No!', although fortunately, patients will rarely be so blunt.

If patients have demonstrated a level of distress, or stated it, then reflecting feelings seems more appropriate. It is often simply a case of inverting the words 'Do you' and saying 'So, you do feel upset', although it is less clumsy to say 'So, it sounds as though you're feeling upset by ...'. The point is that we often ask about emotions, thoughts or experiences which patients have just explained; it seems far better to restate those as a means of demonstrating understanding and empathy.

However, if patients have not demonstrated or stated the feeling or thought, then it might be more appropriate to ask an open question about it, for example 'I'm wondering how you feel about what I've just told you?'.

What does seem important is that nurses consider more fully the purposes behind their questions. Questions can seem intrusive, inquisitive and even impertinent, and may occasionally be asked to serve a nurse's wish for detail rather than to enhance any real understanding of a patient's situation. It is also evident that nurses ask too many questions without stopping to ask patients what questions they may have, and that checking on the areas of doubt, confusion or concern which patients have remains the most sensible, patient-centred starting point.

4. Enabling Patients to Identify the Problem

Of course, there are times when patients do not know what they want from the interaction, or have very vague aims. In these circumstances effective listening and summarizing may lead to the aim emerging, and may encourage patients to consider and 'own' their needs rather than behave as some passive recipient of care to whom things are going to happen.

Spending time getting patients to explore the *experience*, their *feelings* about it, and their *behaviours* is often a useful way of enabling them to see their part in contributing to the situation. This allows patients to see that there are some things within their control. Egan (1994) describes these three components as 'the clarity package' and suggests that, when a client has described all three components they are likely to have a much clearer picture of their current situation.

There are difficulties in enabling patients to identify the problem. Patients may not be ready to look at what is wrong but spend a lot of time complaining that their general practitioner (GP) was slow in sorting out their problems, waiting lists are too long, the hospital doctor looked too young to be trusted and you, the nurse, are useless. It might be tempting to agree for an easy life, or even because we share some of the same opinions! However, this is likely to reinforce the patients' general sense of anger and injustice, confirm their belief that health professionals are either incompetent or not to be trusted and help them to wallow in self-righteous indignation which is ultimately destructive. We will, however, have shown some degree of empathy.

We might, of course, respond by defending the system, criticizing patients or, more probably, feeling inwardly cross and labelling patients as 'difficult'. It is not difficult to imagine the impact of this on individual patients and to acknowledge that the most it will achieve is some relief of frustration for nurses. Of course, it is possible to point out to patients that they seem to be the common denominator in all of this; that is, it might be him or herself, and not all of these other people, who is out of order. This might be accurate, but if delivered badly it will antagonize rather than illuminate the individual.

Helping someone to see the problem clearly is problematic primarily because, unlike the other levels of helping, patients do not normally ask to be challenged. Therefore, nurses are offering interventions for which patients are neither prepared or receptive and, consequently, the interventions need to be clearer, more tentative, and timed with due sensitivity.

Learning Point

- **Challenging** – inviting the patient to view a situation or an experience from a different viewpoint.

The key word is 'inviting', since there is no demand or expectation that the patient will necessarily see things the way the nurse or anyone else does.

Challenging is not one skill, but might be viewed as the impact of a range of skills which lead to that 'Ah, Hah!' moment when the patient says 'I hadn't thought of looking at it that way, but . . .'.

We would like to make two specific statements with respect to challenging difficult or unpopular patients who complain about the system, or seem unduly angry or resentful.

1. Complaints and anger, even when we believe it is unfairly channelled, can be viewed as a *solution* to a problem rather than the problem itself. For example, take the mother on the day unit who is complaining unfairly that nurses are insensitive to her child's needs. She may *need* to feel angry and hostile and find that, unconsciously, hostility is a good defence against the very real fear and anxiety she has about her child's health (getting angry often mobilizes our energy and resources whereas fear can lead to feelings of powerlessness).

Therefore, our starting point would be to attempt to empathize with the mother and communicate some understanding of how she sees the situation, in as non-defensive a way as we could. This takes us back to Level 3 helping. From that base of mutual understanding and trust it might be possible to invite the woman to look at the accuracy of what she is saying and consider an alternative viewpoint. This sense of understanding, coupled with a belief that the nurse is on her side, is vital if the woman is to consider that she may not be being wholly fair or feel encouraged to talk about the concerns which are really troubling her.

2. The challenge should be aimed at helping patients to understand or explore their situation better, and is not designed to 'set them straight'. Therefore, if patients' anger, hostility or misinformation might get in the way of responding to treatment or carrying out postoperative instructions, then it seems necessary to spend some time trying:

- to understand what is going on for individual patients
- helping them to consider the evidence and the helpfulness or otherwise of their current way of viewing things.

However difficult they may be for nurses to accept, if patients' views and emotions are not likely to interfere with treatment, then a decision might be made to leave well alone. Challenging is not easy for a number of reasons:

- It takes a certain amount of courage – patients might be irritated if it is not said in the right way.
- Patients may be hurt and that is not what nurses do.
- It sounds like a complex skill and nurses may not feel able.
- Time is short, it's not worth the effort and patients won't listen anyway.
- I wouldn't like someone challenging me.

Reflection Points

Consider a recent occasion when you dealt with a patient who you considered to be difficult, or blaming or complaining unjustly.

- How did you manage the situation?
- What do you imagine the patient might have been feeling, or trying to convey?
- If you were to return to the situation, what might you say in an attempt to encourage the patient to look at their own behaviour afresh?
- What might stop you?

Yet we would argue that there are times when a degree of assertion is necessary in our dealings with others and that challenging can be seen as respectful of the other person – we are acknowledging that they are tough enough to listen to us and still come to their own conclusions without the world falling apart.

5. Helping the Patient to Manage the Problem

Definitions of counselling often seem rather vague and it could be argued that the one below is no exception. None the less it is a recent attempt to encapsulate the key elements of counselling and demonstrates some of the complexities inherent in counselling such as the wide range and depth of issues that may be addressed. The rest of the code goes on to explore the counselling relationship and indicate that counselling is a skilled and ethical activity.

It is not our intention to describe a counselling model or theory in detail here. We would rather raise some of the issues relating to whether to or when to counsel in day surgery units. If you are interested in counselling we direct you to the reference section at the end of the chapter.

There are a wide variety of views about the desirability of providing counselling facilities for patients which fall within a range from 'We don't have the time to talk to patients, let alone counsel them!' to 'It's an important part of the job that we all do anyway'. Whichever view is taken it is indisputable that patients coming to the unit will have a wide variety of emotional responses to their physical problems and the need for medical intervention, which may include anxiety states, depression and loss or the triggering of previously controlled psychological problems. These are frequently managed without the assistance or even the knowledge of the nursing staff

Learning Point

- **Counselling** – 'The overall aim of counselling is to provide an opportunity for the client to work towards living in a more satisfying and resourceful way . . . . Counselling may be concerned with developmental issues, addressing and resolving specific problems, making decisions, coping with crisis, developing personal insight and knowledge, working through feelings of inner conflict or improving relationships with others' (BAC 1993).

but there are occasions when the patient seeks direct assistance for an issue, or nursing staff identify it through skilled listening and responding.

None the less, whether nurses choose to counsel or not, it seems vital that both parties are clear about the nature of help that is being offered (e.g. nurses may continue to provide a listening ear while someone else provides counselling), and that patients are encouraged to develop their own support network. A useful question we have found in this context is to ask 'If I were not around, who else would you be talking to?'. This can remove some of the pressure or arrogance that may be felt at being the only person supporting someone, and can help patients to develop their own support and minimize both dependency and isolation.

Therefore, it is not essential that all nurses are willing and able to counsel all patients, but we would argue that it *is* desirable that each unit decides whether to provide the facility of counselling for patients or whether it decides that all patients are referred elsewhere to have their longer-term psychological needs met. This brings us back to being able to make an adequate assessment of patients' needs and have an available source for referral.

The general view of staff is that counselling is not wholly appropriate for day surgery patients; '... it's more a case of listening to their worries, understanding and reassuring them'. But it appears that it is often provided in an informal manner for the 'treatments'. So, patients returning to a unit for chemotherapy (if the unit undertakes such treatments) are often seen as in need of counselling and support. This is probably because a relationship is beginning to develop, the time becomes available to listen to the patient and the nurse is seen as the ideal person to help solve problems. Lewis (1994) comments that the fragmented nature of care in theatre nursing militates against effective communication and it is worth considering whether the organization of care in your unit assists in the development of a nurse–patient relationship or whether it creates difficulties.

However, when nurses say they are counselling they need to be clear whether they are offering:

- The opportunity for patients to get things off their chest and to have 'a good moan' – which is *Level 3* helping.
- Information, guidance, advice on how to manage treatment, side effects, or even the children – which is *Level 2* helping.
- The opportunity for patients to identify their current concerns, explore what they really want and identify their own way of getting what they want. This may be about the 'big' issues in their life or it may be about the immediate issues such as managing nausea or coping with lethargy at a particular point in the day – this is *Level 5* helping.

Our issue here is not that one level is necessarily better than another – they all have their strengths and limitations and the choice of which level to use should be determined by the patient's need – but that nurses should be clear about what it is that they are offering and be confident that the unit is prepared to support the time spent with patients at that level.

It could be argued that giving guidance and advice is the quickest, most cost-effective method of providing health education and that patients expect nothing less of highly trained health professionals. Therefore, Level 2 help would seem to have its merits. Equally, there are those who would say that Level 5 help is far more powerful since patients have identified their own issues, goals and solutions from within their own frame of reference and that change is likely to be more permanent and lasting. Patients are also empowered and less likely to become dependent consumers.

When looking at Level 5 helping it is perhaps worth attempting to distinguish between counselling and using counselling skills since the differences are subtle yet important. In 1989, The British Association of Counselling made the following declaration:

> Only when both the user and the recipient explicitly contract to enter into a counselling relationship does it cease to be 'using counselling skills' and become 'counselling'. (BAC 1989)

Therefore, in the majority of nursing situations nurses will be using *counselling skills* when helping another individual to problem solve a particular situation. No matter how skilled nurses are, what they are providing can be viewed as an enhancement to their normal role, and may be seen by themselves, their patients and the organization as a part of their normal working role as a nurse.

For us, *counselling* is a service provided explicitly and clearly for an individual who sees the helper as a counsellor. Counsellors normally have specific skills, training and recognized expertise and it will be seen by all parties that what is being provided is different from the usual service provided by nurses. The essential difference between the two is the contract between helper and patient. When using counselling skills it is possible to slip into the activity as a natural part of what the nurse does, although we would recommend that checking out with patients that this is what they want is highly desirable. The person who takes on the role of counsellor will usually have a more explicit contract regarding boundaries and the purposes of the interview.

Ultimately, the choice of approach will be determined by unit policy and resources, individual nurse's level of confidence in their skills and by individual patient's needs. It would be a shame if nurses continue only to offer one sort of help because that is all they have been trained in or feel confident in without fully considering the variety of needs which patients may be expressing.

Summary

It should be apparent that the boundaries of support are not clear and that nurses need to negotiate, contract and clarify the support on offer to meet their patients' needs. It is also apparent that the demands on nurses' time can be infinite. Identifying which level of help patients require can be a relatively simple task, although it is worth emphasizing that patients may well want to ventilate, receive some information and work out solutions to a problem in one 5-minute interaction. On the whole, the sensible way to identify what the patients want is to ask them; they just might tell us!

Organizations also have a responsibility to their patients and staff to identify clearly what is being offered, by whom, and under what terms, since providing quality support is extremely time consuming yet rarely considered when reviewing staffing establishments. We would argue that supporting patients is a vital part of the role of the nurse in contemporary day surgery; a role that requires supervision, support and time to perform it effectively and efficiently to the satisfaction of the greatest number of people. This means that nurses can and should demand support of their managers in ensuring that high-quality interpersonal helping can be provided, rather than using lack of resources as a reason for not spending sufficient time with patients.

Key Points

- The literature on nurse–patient communication suggests that it could be better.
- Nurses sometimes struggle to identify what level of help patients actually want from them.
- Five Levels of Helping are offered as a framework.
- The decision on which level to offer should be made in conjunction with the patient.
- Information-giving is a vital part of day surgery provision and is generally valued but nurses are seldom told how best to do this – it is assumed we can all do it naturally.
- Communication skills can be learnt and developed.
- Counselling and the use of counselling skills are two discrete activities.
- Listening to the patient is the starting point in all situations. It is the base from which all other approaches are developed.
- Challenging may be the most difficult because the patient has not requested it and the nurse may be less skilled at effectively challenging.
- The effective use of interpersonal skills requires motivation to do so, the necessary skills and training, time and the support of the organization. It is a matter for the whole culture of the unit rather than the interest or aptitude of one or two individuals.

Recommended Reading

Egan, G. (1994) **The Skilled Helper** (Fifth Edition) Belmont, California: Brooks Cole

Possibly the most widely taught model of counselling with three distinct merits. First, it has similarities to the nursing process – the three stages are I, What is the problem? II, What do you want? (Goals) III, How are you going to get there? (Action Planning). Second, it is a very practical model which can apply to relatively long-term counselling but also to very short-term use of counselling skills. Third, it has stood the test of time.

Chapters 8 and 9 focus on challenging and help expand on Level 4 skills to enable problem identification

Tschudin, V. (1995) **Counselling Skills for Nurses** (Fourth Edition) London: Baillière Tindall

Like Egan's book this has stood the test of time but the author's application of skills to a UK nursing setting adds credence to her insightful observations

References

Alcock, P. (1986) **Preoperative information and visits promote recovery of patients.** *British Journal of Theatre Nursing* **July**: 17–18.

Ashworth, P. (1980) **Care to communicate**. London: RCN.

Audit Commission (1991) **Measuring quality: The patients view of day surgery.** London: HMSO.

Avis, M. (1992) **Silent partners: patients' views about choice and decision making in a day unit.** *British Journal of Theatre Nursing* **2**(7): 8–11.

Bond, S. (1983) **Nurses communication with cancer patients**. In Wilson Barnett, J. (Ed) *Nursing Research.* Chichester: Wiley.

Boore, J. R. P. (1978) **Prescription for recovery.** London: RCN.

Bowling, A. (1992) **Assessing health needs and measuring patient satisfaction.** *Nursing Times* **88**(31): 31–34.

Brammer, L. (1993) **The Helping Relationship** (Fifth Edition). London: Prentice Hall.

British Association of Counselling (BAC) (1989) **The Code of Ethics and Practice for Counsellors.** London: BAC.

British Association of Counselling (BAC) (1993) **The Code of Ethics and Practice for Counsellors.** London: BAC.

Burnard, P. and Morrison, P. (1989) **What is an interpersonally skilled person? A repertory grid account of professional nurses' views.** *Nurse Education Today* **9**: 384–391.

Egan, G. (1994) **The Skilled Helper** (Fifth Edition). Belmont, California: Brooks Cole.

Faulkner, A. (1981) **Aye, there's the rub.** *Nursing Times* 19 Feb. 332–336.

Gott, M. (1984) **Learning nursing; a study of the effectiveness and relevance of teaching during student nurse introductory course.** London: RCN.

Hathaway, D. (1986) **Effect of preoperative instruction on post operative outcomes: a meta-analysis.** *Nursing Research* **35**(5): 269–275.

Hayward, J. (1975) **Information: A prescription against pain.** London: RCN.

Helman, C. (1990) **Culture, Health & Illness** (Second Edition). Oxford: Butterworth Heinemann.

Johnson, G. (1990) **Pre-op visits; why they don't happen.** *Nursing* **19**: 24–27.

Lewis, M. (1994) **Communication in theatres.** *Surgical Nurse* **7**: 27–29.

Macleod-Clark, J. (1981) **Communication in nursing.** *Nursing Times* Jan 1: 12–18.

Macleod-Clark, J. (1984) **Verbal communication in nursing**. In Faulkner, A. (Ed) *Recent Advances in Nursing.* London: Churchill Livingstone.

Menzies, I. (1960) **A case study in the functioning of social systems as a defence against anxiety.** London: Tavistock Institute of Human Relations.

Murphy, S. J. (1994) **Preoperative assessment for day surgery.** *Surgical Nurse* **7**(3): 6–9.

Rogers, C. (1961) **On Becoming a Person.** London: Constable.

Stockwell, F. (1972) **The unpopular patient.** London: RCN.

Swindale, J. E. (1989) **The nurses role in giving preoperative information to reduce anxiety in patients admitted to hospital from elective minor surgery.** *Journal of Advanced Nursing* **14**: 899–905.

Tschudin, V. (1995) **Counselling Skills for Nurses.** (Fourth Edition). London: Baillière Tindall.

Wilson, T. (1996) **Levels of helping: a framework to assist tutors in providing tutorial support at the level students want and need.** *Nurse Education Today* **16**: 270–273.

Wright, H. (1991) **The patient, the nurse, his life and her mother: psychodynamic influences in nurse education and practice.** *Psychoanalytic Psychotherapy* **5**(2): 139–149.

Chapter 5 Screening and selection

Overview

Developing means of accurately assessing the suitability of all patients for general anaesthesia and surgery is continuing to attract attention in the current medical and nursing press. As part of the overall reduction in length of hospital stay, it is now common practice for inpatients to be admitted on the day of surgery, so the need to establish fitness prior to this time has become a major concern. The same clearly applies to those patients having day surgery. This chapter therefore looks at the development of pre-admission selection, assessment and preparation of patients within the context of day surgery. Clearly, any protocols must take account of psycho-social factors as well as physical status. It is also important to address the specific needs of differing patient groups, especially children and the elderly. In this chapter we explore the growth and organization of pre-assessment clinics and the pivotal role of the day surgery nurse in their development, outlining the essential quality and safety standards involved and the need for multidisciplinary decision-making.

Future inclusion of older and potentially less fit patients for day surgery and the growing adoption of 'one-stop' approaches to the organization of pre-admission assessment may require that more nurses develop further skills in assessing patients' cardiovascular and respiratory status. This chapter therefore also looks at the rationales for the more commonly used clinical preselection screening procedures of electrocardiography and spirometry.

Chapter Focus

- Selection of procedures for day surgery
- Selection criteria
  - general medical
  - anaesthetic
  - social
- Pre-operative screening
- Nurse-led pre-admission assessment

Introduction

The success of national day surgery initiatives and the quality of individual patient experiences hinges upon the careful selection of procedures deemed suitable for day surgery *and* the selection of patients to undergo these procedures.

Further increase both in numbers and complexity of day surgery cases clearly requires a systematic means of selecting and screening patients in order to maximize the potential of the service. However, the NHS Management Executive (1993) emphasizes strongly that the pursuit of higher day surgery percentages should not be undertaken at the expense of sound clinical decision-making and selection of appropriate treatment options for individual patients. Increasing day surgery therefore must not be seen as an end in itself, rather more as a means to achieving a number of different ends, of which, quality of the patient experience is central. Indeed, the Audit Commission (1991) argues that as purchasers are now setting minimum standards within their contracts for day surgery, they are therefore in a position to maintain and improve the quality of patient experience.

Changes in both surgical and anaesthetic procedures have increased the number of patients eligible for day surgery, once more underlining the need for rigorous preoperative selection and assessment. Further, both the Audit Commission (1990) and the Royal College of Surgeons (1992) support nurses taking the lead role in such assessment. Whilst any pre-admission assessment must achieve the safe and appropriate selection of patients from both clinical and psycho-social perspectives, nurses should also make the most of the opportunity that pre-admission assessment provides to begin to develop relationships with patients. Such relationships can have positive and measurable effects on patients' experience of day surgery, and therefore the role of the nurse in this process is pivotal.

Selection of Procedures

As outlined in Chapter 1, quite a large number of surgeons and anaesthetists were resistant initially to developing day surgery services. Historically, it appears that many surgeons came into day surgery almost by default with a clear purpose of reducing their waiting lists when it became apparent that increased inpatient bed space and operating time were not forthcoming (Jarrett 1989). However, it seems that from the surgeons' early experiences of day surgery the benefits quickly became apparent both to themselves, in more efficient use of operating time and reduced cancellations, and to their patients, who genuinely seemed to prefer this option when possible.

Massive changes both in available clinical technology and funding of health services have influenced significantly the development of day surgery practice and subsequently, the selection of procedures. Bridger and Rees (1995) suggest that purchasers are achieving cost savings between 25 and 65% through the development of procedure-specific day surgery contracts with providers. Whilst it is interesting to observe the ongoing media debate surrounding the increase in 'keyhole' or minimal access surgery (MAS), it does raise some important concerns. Unfortunately for the health professionals, both the positive aspects to these developments and the sometimes quite sensationalist headlines about lack of training and questions about safety are often discussed in the context of *day surgery*. On occasion, the style of the presentation could lead an observer to perceive these two issues as one and the same; that is, day surgery is synonymous with minimal access surgery. But the reality is often very different.

Laparoscopic surgical techniques and use of laser technology have undoubtedly reduced many of the undesirable effects of surgery, improved the experience for patients and made some complex procedures *possible* as day cases. But whilst there is little doubt that MAS approaches will continue to develop for the benefit of many, it is also important to acknowledge the very real concerns surrounding their effectiveness and associated levels of clinical competence and training. Bloor and Maynard (1994) believe that the lack of regulation of such technological growth is fundamentally wrong and argue that MAS techniques should be subject to the same rigorous clinical and economical evaluation measures that are currently applied to pharmaceutical products. The evolution in such products, especially in the fields of anaesthesia and pain control, have been just as significant in creating both the present and future potential for day surgery. The development of intravenous anaesthetic agents such as *propofol* is but one example. This is not the cheapest option, but propofol does help patients enjoy a rapid and more clear-headed recovery in addition to a substantially reduced likelihood of postoperative nausea and vomiting. This example demonstrates the role of *economic* evaluation in clinical decision-making.

Commissioners keen to achieve the best outcomes for patients are likely to want to contract for the MAS option. But targets or thresholds will not be achieved through contracts that stipulate that all inguinal hernia repairs are to be carried out laparoscopically and, furthermore, as day cases. There will always be the need for inpatient options for surgery now readily recognized as a day case procedure. Similarly, setting national targets for day surgery seems inappropriate as this approach clearly fails to take account of local needs and practises. According to the NHS Management Executive (1993), increases in numbers of minor and intermediate procedures should be brought about by local agreements between purchasers and providers, that is doing 'more of the same', whilst looking to widen the present anaesthetic criteria. But however contracting proceeds, or how the surgery is carried out, the ability to identify those patients at risk remains paramount.

Most surgical specialties now include a large number of procedures that are able to be undertaken on a day surgery basis, and one of the most important criteria is *operating time*. Clearly, the longer an operation takes to perform, the more anaesthesia will be required and the patient will need longer to recover. Also, fewer numbers will be able to be accommodated on one list, which may be counterproductive. Offering a broad guide, The Royal College of Surgeons (1992) initially suggested that day case procedures should last no longer than 60 min, with an optimum of 30–45 min. However, few patients with the same condition share identical characteristics, so simple categories of procedure are not sufficient. For example, inguinal hernia repair is identified as one of the standard day case operative procedures, but consideration must be given at initial outpatient consultation to another important criterion: *the size and complexity of individual patient's pathology.*

With these considerations in mind, general surgical procedures such as varicose vein surgery, breast lump excision, hernia repair and haemorrhoidectomy are undertaken routinely on a day case basis. Gynaecological procedures include D & C (though the efficacy of this particular procedure is being questioned), diagnostic laparoscopy, hysteroscopy, laparascopic sterilization and termination of pregnancy. Procedures within the fields of orthopaedics, ear, nose and throat (ENT), ophthalmics and genito-urinary surgery make up the Audit Commission's (1990) original 'basket of procedures' (see Chapter 1), and are routinely carried out as day cases. The list is expanding and will continue to do so, less now as a result of simple enthusiasm and more in response to local needs, growth in technology and expertise and local improvements in organization and provision. Much of the success depends on rigorous pre-admission assessment.

Selection of Patients

So what exactly is pre-admission assessment and what should it seek to achieve? Markanday and Platzer (1994) define pre-assessment as:

> a pre-admission interview between nurse and patient in which the patient is assessed for his or her physical, psychological and social suitability to have their surgery performed as a day case. It is also a time during which the patient is psychologically prepared for the operation and given pre-operative instructions to follow and postoperative advice so that he or she can plan for their discharge.

Most providers agree that the prime focus of any pre-assessment programme should be the safe selection of patients for surgical procedures; selection that is based on agreed social and general medical criteria. Patients can also be provided with more in-depth information about their forthcoming surgery and aftercare and have any questions answered. In addition, attendance at a pre-assessment clinic or facility provides patients and their relatives with the opportunity to familiarize themselves with the day surgery unit and to meet some of the staff who will be involved in caring for them; this is especially important for children and their parents. Another important, yet often underestimated, aspect of pre-admission assessment is that it provides an ideal opportunity for nursing staff to begin to build relationships with patients that in turn may go some way to reduce the incidence of pre-operative anxiety. It is also probably true that only when such relationships are built can nurses use this pre-admission time for important health-related teaching (Dobson 1992, Ewles & Simnett 1992). This final point is obviously based on an assumption that it is the day surgery unit nurses who will undertake such assessment, and that need not be the case (see section on Methods of organizing pre-admission assessment later in this chapter).

This is beginning to look like quite a task for nursing staff to achieve, given the other aspects of their role. It is also potentially quite an ordeal for patients to go through, especially if they are still trying to come to terms with the prospect of surgery. On these two counts, it would be tempting to reduce the pre-admission assessment to the minimum. But, as Farrelly and Lakeman (1993) point out, patient education in itself is a rather complex activity that involves a lot more than the giving and receiving of information.

An insightful indication of the potential for education and support and the nursing communication, teaching and organizational skills required is provided by Dutton (1994). She argues that the example of patients undergoing termination of pregnancy clearly illustrates the need for a sensitive, yet comprehensive approach to pre-admission assessment and education. Whilst the organization of pre-admission assessment facilities varies enormously from one unit to the next in this country, there does appear to be greater consensus in terms of purpose. According to Vijay *et al.* (1995) pre-admission assessment allows for confirmation of patients' suitability for surgery, and the provision of written and verbal information regarding procedures. In addition, patients and their relatives have the opportunity to look around the unit if they so wish. This could be particularly important for parents with children.

Confirmation of Suitability

> Quite apart from the suitability of the type of operation, selection for day surgical treatment requires an assessment of the patient's health and social circumstances (Royal College of Surgeons 1992).

Therefore, the three fundamental variables to be addressed at pre-admission assessment are:

- general medical status
- social circumstances
- anaesthetic fitness.

General Medical Status

The principal framework for assessing patients' general medical suitability for day case surgery is provided by the American Society of Anaesthesiologists (ASA 1991). Their classification organizes all surgical patients into one of five classes of physical fitness (Box 5.1).

The Royal College of Surgeons (1992) suggest that as a rule, only patients in ASA Class 1 (those who are normally fit and well) and Class 2 (those with mild, but controlled disease) are suitable for day surgery. They further suggest that obese patients with a body mass index (BMI – calculated by dividing unclothed weight in kilograms by height in metres^2) greater than 30 should also be excluded and any upper age limit introduced to be based on biological, rather than chronological age. As Vijay *et al.* (1995) point out, excluding patients on the grounds of age presents some considerable difficulties when operating in a geographical area where the elderly are the predominant members. Adopting a more rational approach will mean that more elderly and therefore potentially less fit patients in Classes 3 and 4 are now being included for specific (especially urological) procedures. Demographic changes and increased targets will no doubt see more and more elderly people having surgical procedures on a day case basis. With the actual and potential incidence of cardiovascular and respiratory diseases being much higher in the elderly groups, and the potential for reduced social support much less, the physical and psychosocial

Box 5.1 Classification of surgical patients (adapted from ASA 1991)

Class 1
Absence of organic, physiological, biochemical or psychiatric disturbance.

Class 2
Mild to moderate systemic disturbance, caused either by condition to be treated surgically or another disease process; e.g. mild diabetes or anaemia, controlled essential hypertension. Extremes of age (neonate or 80–90 years) even without discernible disease, extreme obesity and chronic bronchitis can be placed in this category.

Class 3
Severe systemic disease, e.g. organic heart disease, severe diabetes with vascular complications, moderate to severe respiratory insufficiency, angina, or old (> 6 months) myocardial infarction.

Class 4
Severe, life-threatening disturbances which may not be corrrectable by planned surgical intervention, e.g. unstable angina, marked cardiac, pulmonary, hepatic, renal or endocrine insufficiency.

Class 5
Collapsed patient who has little chance of survival but is submitted to surgery in desparation, often as a resuscitative measure with little or no anaesthesia, e.g. leaking or ruptured aortic aneurysm, cerebral trauma with rising intracranial pressure.

impacts of a major shift in approach to surgical management in this group of patients warrants investigation. For a résumé of pre-admission assessment from an anaesthetist's perspective, please see Chapter 8.

Although the ASA classification has been in use since the early 1960s, there is some evidence to suggest that inconsistencies in interpretation of the classes by anaesthetists is occurring in practice (Haynes & Awler 1995) and that similar anomalies occur between different grades and levels of experience of surgical staff (NHSME Value for Money Unit 1991). This latter study reported that some junior doctors were clearly not aware that such a classification even existed, and at that time some 10% of patients arriving for day surgery were found to be unsuitable for general anaesthetic. It is also interesting that some of the anaesthetists taking part in this study believed that their surgeon colleagues tended to ignore social and general medical indicators of suitability, basing their decision solely on the specific condition requiring surgical intervention.

As a result, the NHS Management Executive recommended that hospitals review their practices regarding assessment of patients for general anaesthetic as day cases, also suggesting that a busy outpatient department might not represent the ideal environment for such an assessment to take place.

Social Circumstances

The effects of general anaesthesia on concentration, co-ordination and judgement are well known. It is vital that all patients undergoing day surgery are accompanied home (they *must not* be allowed to drive) and have arranged for an adult to be present with them for the first 24 h following their operation. The patient's home conditions must be sufficient to allow them to recover in comfort; they should have access to a telephone in case of emergencies and should live within an hour's journey from the hospital (Royal College of Surgeons 1992). The point about adequate housing conditions is fraught with difficulties. Who makes the judgement about adequacy? Generally, it appears that housing is assumed adequate if there is an inside toilet; that is, the patient will not have to walk outside to use it. Many two-storey houses have their toilet on the ground floor, which still entails a walk; comfort is surely dependent on other factors, and is essentially a subjective judgement. For example, what of the travelling families who live in caravans? Are they to be automatically excluded? It is perhaps too easy to make assumptions about their lifestyle and decide that such conditions are inadequate for postoperative recovery. Assessment protocols must have room for individual cases and decisions should be made using clinical judgement, not value judgement.

Anaesthetic Fitness

In addition to information about social and domestic circumstances and general medical fitness, it is also important to establish present fitness for general anaesthetic. Questions are routinely asked about known allergies, use of prescription and non-prescription medication and consumption of alcohol and tobacco; all provide significant information for anaesthetic assessment. In addition, common assessment measures used are height, weight and BMI, blood-pressure recording and routine urinalysis; some or all of these may be utilized on your unit. (The decision to include such measures should be based on multidisciplinary discussion of available evidence and local needs, not accepted custom and practice.)

In the light of evidence of substantial errors in recordings and established inaccuracies associated with manual sphygmomanometers (Draper 1987), it is vital that blood pressures are recorded using an electronic device. The Royal College of Surgeons (1992) suggest that older patients (as low as 50 years in some units) may require similar pre-operative investigation to those undergoing surgery as inpatients. This could include chest X-ray, electrocardiography (ECG), full blood count and serum urea and electrolyte estimation. It is of note that the efficacy of routine ECG recording is being increasingly questioned (Edwards & Riley 1994). In addition, Callaghan *et al.* (1995) investigated the use of preoperative ECG and found that only 7% of patients aged over 50 years with no risk factors had an abnormal ECG. They argue that the presence of cardiac disease or risk factors for cardiac disease should be the criteria for utilization of preoperative ECG, not chronological age.

Patients with asthma who do not routinely take steroids or others with a past history of respiratory insufficiency may also require assessment of their pulmonary function. Such investigations, though deemed by many to be standard pre-operative measures, must be subjected to evaluation both in terms of unit costs and the use of nursing and patients' time. Davies and Ogg (1993) advocate the minimum use of pre-operative investigations, arguing that only patients over 75 years with a significant medical history should have routine ECG, chest X-ray, etc. The importance of negotiation between the clinical director and surgeons and anaesthetists is two-fold. First, to establish rational pre-operative assessment protocols for specific patient groups in day surgery and second to determine locally agreed, non-ambiguous inclusion and exclusion criteria.

Possible Pre-operative Assessment Measures

Biochemistry

Patients with suspected impairment of renal filtration, absorption and excretion functions, for example as a result of hypertension, will have changes in plasma concentrations of electrolytes and metabolites. Estimation of serum urea and electrolytes will indicate the presence/extent of renal dysfunction. However, it is worth noting that over 50% of renal function has to be lost before changes will be seen in the urea and creatinine concentrations. Again, this underlines the importance of evaluation of the use of biochemistry. The normal values (Royle & Walsh 1992) are outlined below:

Urea	2.9–8.9 mmol l^{-1}
Creatinine	60–120 mmol l^{-1}
Uric acid	0.22–0.48 mmol l^{-1}
Sodium	135–145 mmol l^{-1}
Potassium	3.5–5.5 mmol l^{-1}
Magnesium	0.8–1.3 mmol l^{-1}
Phosphate	0.8–1.5 mmol l^{-1}
Chlorine	100–106 mmol l^{-1}
Calcium	2.2–2.6 mmol l^{-1}
Bicarbonate	24–28 mmol l^{-1}

Haematology

This involves a full blood count for estimation of haemoglobin, leucocytes, platelets and haematocrit. This is likely to be requested in patients with a history of excessive blood loss and suspected anaemia, for example women with menorrhagia. The haemoglobin concentration is the value of most interest and may be estimated by ward-based techniques if necessary. The minimum level suitable for day case anaesthesia requires local discussion but will be around 9–10 g dl^{-1}. Normal values are as follows (Royle & Walsh 1992):

Haemoglobin	Males 14-18 g dl^{-1}	(8.1–11.2 mmol l^{-1})
	Females 12–16 g dl^{-1}	(7.4–9.9 mmol l^{-1})
Leucocytes	4.0–11.0 × 10^9 l^{-1}	
Thrombocytes	150–400 × 10^9 l^{-1}	
Haematocrit	Males 40–50%	
	Females 37–47%	

Radiology

The use of chest X-ray provides a relatively simple means of identifying chest structure and possible lesions, though the value of routine chest X-ray is questionable (RCR 1989). This investigation is more commonly carried out in older patients with a history of respiratory disease.

Electrocardiography (ECG)

ECG records the electrical activities of the heart and remains the most commonly used means of detecting cardiac ischaemia and arrhythmias. In a 12-lead ECG, electrodes are placed on the limbs and anterior chest wall. Upward deflections are seen when an impulse is travelling towards an electrode and downwards as the impulse travels away (Hatfield & Tronson 1992). An ECG tracing (Fig. 5.1) has the following components:

- *P wave* – contraction of the atria – is absent in atrial fibrillation
- *QRS complex* – onset of ventricular contraction – if notched or widened, is usually indicative of ventricular muscle damage, past or present
- *ST segment* – continuation of ventricular contraction – if depressed or inverted, again indicative of ventricular muscle damage
- *T wave* – recovery phase following ventricular contraction – if flattened, peaked or inverted – muscle damage

According to Hatfield and Tronson (1992), the following questions should be determined when reading and interpreting an ECG:

- establish the heart rate
- establish if rhythm is normal
- establish the presence of a P wave
- establish if QRS complex is normal
- if not, is the rhythm dangerous and does it need treatment?

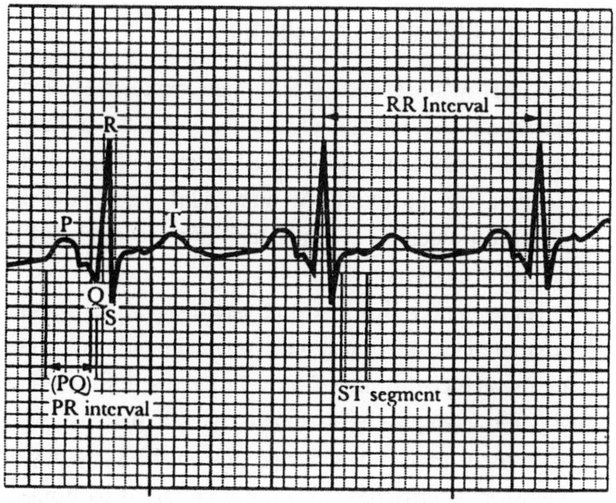

Figure 5.1 Normal ECG trace

Spirometry

These investigations assess the movement of air into and out of the lungs and as such are valuable in identifying potential respiratory difficulties pre-operatively. Table 5.1 summarizes the different lung function measures.

Table 5.1 Different lung function measures (adapted from Royle & Walsh 1992)

Test	Symbol	Description	Comments
Vital capacity	VC	The maximal volume of air exhaled following a maximal inspiration (norm = 3500–5000 ml)	↓ in restrictive airway disease because of limited lung expansion. In obstructive airways disease the total lung capacity is ↑ but VC may be ↓ due to air trapping with ↑ residual volume
Tidal volume	V_T	The volume of air exhaled following a normal breath (norm = 450–750 ml)	
Forced vital capacity	FVC	The maximal volume of air that can be forcibly and rapidly exhaled following a maximal inspiration	↓ in obstructive airways disease due to air trapping
Timed vital capacity	FEV_T	The percentage of vital capacity that can be expelled after 1, 2 and 3 s (FEV_1, FEV_2 and FEV_3) Norm = 80, 90 & 95% respectively)	↓ in obstructive airways disease because of ↑ airway resistance; usually normal in restrictive airway disease
Maximal voluntary ventilation	MVV	The maximal volume of air that can be breathed in a given time interval (norm = 40–70 breaths per minute breathing half VC each breath)	Least accurate of timed breathing tests, but useful indicator of exercise tolerance
Residual volume	RV	The volume of gas remaining in the lungs at the end of a maximal expiration (norm = 25–40% of total lung capacity, e.g. 1500 ml)	↑ in obstructive airways disease
Functional residual capacity	FRC	The volume of air remaining in the lungs after a passive exhalation in normal breathing (normal = about 3000 ml)	↑ in obstructive airways disease

Methods of Organizing Pre-admission Assessment

It is worthwhile spending some time exploring the various organizational options that exist and examining some of the advantages and disadvantages associated with each. From the available, yet largely anecdotal, literature a number of approaches to organizing pre-admission assessment facilities can be found. An important factor in this debate appears to be whether the pre-admission assessment clinic facilities are intended for all surgical patients or just for those requiring day surgery.

There is no right or wrong way to go about pre-admission assessment. However, there are a number of factors that should be considered when planning such a service in order that resources are used efficiently and effectively and disruption to patients' lives is kept to a minimum. It should not, for example, be assumed that all patients would prefer to have all investigations and assessment procedures carried out on the same day as their consultation. (The development of 'one-stop' approaches, apparently preferred by nurses is based on the assumption that patients would prefer this option – see Bottrill 1994). This could particularly apply (though not exclusively) to some elderly patients relying on others for transport and support and to parents with younger children for whom a stay in outpatients can be a particularly wearing experience. Similarly, spending some time in a busy outpatient department would soon reveal to planners the fatigue associated with simply waiting to see their surgeon. Opportunities for conversations can be rather limited, reading material is often out of date and inappropriate. When they finally do get to see the consultant and are told that they require surgery, it is not unreasonable that some may prefer just to go home. Some patients will elect to discuss their surgery with their family and friends before undergoing pre-operative assessment and investigation. After all, this too is likely to involve more waiting.

It is in some ways rather arrogant to presume that to have everything done on one day will be best for patients, as it is often based on the premise that patients have nothing better to do. As discussed in Chapter 3, people place different degrees of importance on their health and after a long and frustrating wait in outpatients (or even a short one), followed by a 3.5-min consultation, other activities of life such as shopping or childcare may then rightfully assume priority. Whilst this observation is neither new or applicable to all patients attending outpatients, maybe the implications for patients rights does need to be made more explicit. Patients may then really be given the choice about having pre-admission assessment completed on the same day or returning at a later date. Two commonly utilized approaches are outlined below:

Separate Clinic within Outpatient Department

This approach consists of geographically siting the assessment facilities within the outpatient department, but managing them as separate clinics. Some new integrated day units are adjacent to outpatients (Bottrill 1994), which is probably the ideal. Patients are referred by standard proforma by the surgeon for assessment that same day or for a subsequent appointment, depending on patient's preference. The clinics are run by nursing staff, with or without clerical support, depending on numbers, and often with support when needed for anaesthetic decisions from the duty anaesthetist or junior house officer. Any pre-operative investigations such as X-rays and blood tests can be arranged through normal outpatient protocols.

Box 5.2 Advantages and disadvantages of locating pre-admission assessment facilities in OPD

Advantages

- Ease of referral; the clinic's close proximity to the area of initial consultation means that patients who do not meet all required criteria can be referred back to the surgeon or placed on the inpatient waiting list.
- Running the clinic in outpatients also makes it easier for patients to be seen on that same day with minimal disruption and delay.
- Nurses who have undergone special preparation and training run the clinics, do not have the pressure of other role requirements and therefore have more opportunities to organize specific teaching and health promotion sessions.

Disadvantages

- Time rarely allows for re-referral back to the surgeon.
- Minimal disruption and delay is more for the benefit of assessment staff than patients.
- Unless the day unit is adjacent to the clinic, a separate visit may need to be arranged to familiarize patients with the area, if they so wish.
- Nurses working on the day unit do not have the opportunity to meet any of their patients until the day of admission.
- Potential for important individual patient information 'getting lost' unless reliable means of documentation used.

Separate Facility within the Day Surgery Unit

This appears to be the most common approach adopted within self-contained day surgery units at the present time. Nurses from the day surgery unit undertake all pre-admission assessments following specific preparation and training; this may entail developing skills in recording and interpreting spirometry and ECG. Patients are referred to the unit directly from outpatients for assessment either on that day or at a later date.

Box 5.3 Advantages and disadvantages of integrating pre-admission assessment facilities in day surgery units

Advantages

- Nurses familiar with specific selection criteria do all assessments.
- Ensures that all nurses have the opportunity to acquire necessary skills, thereby facilitating staff development.
- Allows for flexibility in timing of assessments; patients may prefer to return at a later date if they have other commitments.
- Nursing staff skilled and experienced with caring for children can organize special children's sessions where parents and siblings can familiarize themselves with the unit and meet nursing staff to care for them.
- Tours around the unit can be arranged *if patients so wish,* and therefore anxiety related to the unknown can be reduced.
- When organization allows, the nurse who completes the pre-admission assessment may then become the patient's primary or named nurse.

Disadvantages

- Requires special area set aside for purpose of assessment; this may be difficult to achieve when space is at a premium.
- Preparation and training for role requires commitment and support which may not be forthcoming.
- Nurses themselves may not consider that specific skills are required and adopt an 'anyone can do this' approach.
- Requires that one member of staff is always available to complete pre-admission assessment.
- Patients may get lost if not escorted or signs are not clear.

As with the previous approach, the decision should be made on the basis of what constitutes minimal disruption, *from the patient's point of view.* In addition to information about the benefits of having same-day assessment, an accurate and honest indication of further waiting time needs to be given to patients and their relatives.

But there is another more important factor to be considered here. For pre-admission assessment to be effective it needs a 'best by' or 'expiry' date. There appears little point in pre-assessing patients on the same day as their initial outpatient consultation if the date of surgery cannot be booked at the same time. Assessment that takes place 12 months prior to varicose vein surgery (a real example – see Chapter 4) can no longer be regarded as an accurate representation of that person's medical or social circumstances. Simply asking the people to get in touch if anything changes places an unfair responsibility on the patient to judge what is and what is not important; it is the hospital's responsibility to assess safely an individual's suitability for day surgery. In addition, having such a long gap between assessment and surgery also negates any positive effects of the educative/support element of the pre-admission assessment, and makes the time spent by individual nurses appear wasted. Timing of pre-admission assessment must take waiting list times into account and be organized in such a way that ensures that patients are assessed within a month of surgery.

Regardless of specific differences in organization, pre-admission assessment must meet the needs of greatly varying patient groups. Day units that carry out urological procedures, for example, are likely to have large numbers of elderly people to assess who may not be within standard criteria for inclusion; they may be regular attenders but still require anaesthetic assessment. The same day unit may be also carrying out a number of dedicated paediatric lists for different surgical specialties and may involve children attending hospital for the first time accompanied by understandably anxious parents. Norris (1992) cites evidence that mothers on day units are more anxious as they perceive their responsibility for caring for their child to be greater; nurses involved in pre-admission assessment and the protocols they use must be sufficiently sensitive to meet individual needs and to ensure the accurate assessment of these very different groups.

It may be beneficial for these specific groups, and indeed any individual who expresses the need, to split pre-admission assessment into two discrete areas:

- pre-screening and selection measures – always individually completed
- preparation, teaching and support – may include teaching of relaxation techniques (see Chapter 7) and could be done as small group.

Although straightforward in theory, in practice too much attention is often placed on one aspect of pre-admission assessment (selection) at the expense of the other (teaching and support). It almost seems that the name given to the assessment process (pre-screening, pre-assessment, pre-admission assessment and patient education are but a few) dictates the manner in which it will proceed. More explicit recognition of the two equally important aspects of pre-admission assessment would improve both nurses' and patients' experience. Separating the two areas could also mean that some patients need only attend one session or both, depending on individual circumstances. The sessions could be further tailored towards the needs of children, women, the elderly, first-time attenders, etc. Ideally, the same nursing staff should be involved.

Box 5.4 Research study

In a Canadian study, Ellerton and Merriam (1994) evaluated the use of a pre-admission assessment programme for children aged between 3 and 15 years. The children were all anaesthetically suitable for day surgery. The focus of the programme, which took place on five consecutive Saturdays, was on psychological preparation of children about to undergo day surgery and their families. Of the 75 families in the study, 22 underwent the pre-operative programme which included a videotape of one real family's experience of day surgery, play and a tour of the unit. The remaining 53 families did not come for a number of reasons (distance from the hospital was the most common), but were willing to take part in the study.

On the day of surgery, a semi-structure interview assessed both parental and child anxiety for all 75 families on admission to the unit, in the operating room waiting area and at discharge. Child anxiety was measured using a scale of seven faces, each indicating different experiences and parental anxiety was assessed using a visual analogue scale. The results indicate that 'attendance at the preparation programme was associated with lower levels of anxiety in both parents and children . . . and the association was strongest in the period immediately before the child's surgery'. It was also of note that children of parents with hospital experience and the parents themselves were more anxious immediately prior to surgery than first-time attenders. The authors conclude that the programme provides valuable information and support, and that experience is not always a good teacher (Ellerton & Merriam 1994).

Clearly, this arrangement would require substantial investments in time, training and commitment.

The development of a preparation programme (as separate from assessment) for children is outlined briefly in Box 5.4.

As mentioned earlier, sometimes the time spent on support and health related teaching in a pre-admission assessment programme is less than ideal. The reality of clinical practice places other demands on unit staff so that sometimes the basic safe minimum is completed (screening and selection) and the patients sent on their way armed with leaflets and a lot to think about. But at the same time, the success of pre-admission assessment has increased expectations of it. So, as nurses realize the potential for assessment in terms of improved patient outcomes, the more it grows, it involves an increasing amount of time to complete, and places further pressure on human resources.

Bottrill (1994) describes the introduction of a 'one stop shop' approach to patient selection and assessment (apparently the phrase of the moment) where pre-admission assessment follows initial outpatient consultation in the adjacent day unit. Patients who are deemed suitable, having undergone relevant screening and assessment, are with some degree of choice, given their day of surgery. Bottrill describes typical patient interviews lasting 20–25 min, which allows for full discussion on pre- and postoperative care and for questions to be answered. Commitment to maintaining this level of quality clearly needs to be reflected in staff levels and preparation.

The Pre-admission Assessment Experience

Most of the information necessary to establish general medical and social suitability and some of that required for assessment of anaesthetic fitness can be elicited through a self-completion questionnaire as outlined in Fig. 5.2.

The assessing nurse should give the questionnaire to the patient at the start of the pre-admission assessment, accompanied by a brief explanation of the rationale. In addition, some

Figure 5.2 Pre-admission assessment check list

PRE-ADMISSION ASSESSMENT FOR DAY SURGERY

Maintenance of Air and Circulation

Blood pressure ....
Pulse ....

Have you ever suffered from any of the following:

		YES	NO
1	chest pain on exercise or at night		
2	breathlessness		
3	high blood pressure		
4	heart murmur		
5	heart attack		
6	anaemia or other blood problems		
7	excessive bleeding or bruising		
8	deep venous thrombosis		
9	asthma		
10	fainting easily		

Do you:

		YES	NO
11	smoke		
12	take any medication (tablets, patches, injections, inhalers)		

Maintenance of food and water intake

Height ....
Weight ....
BMI ....

Have you ever suffered from any of the following:

		YES	NO
13	indigestion or heartburn		
14	diabetes		
15	jaundice		

Do you:

		YES	NO
16	drink more than 1½ pints of beer or 3 shorts a day		

Maintenance of Elimination

Urinalysis ....

Have you ever suffered from any of the following:

		YES	NO
17	kidney or urinary trouble		
18	bowel problems		

Figure 5.2 Continued

Prevention of Hazards

Have you ever had:

		YES	NO
19	an allergy to general anaesthetic		
20	a serious illness		
21	allergy or reaction to medicines, Elastoplast, or metals		
22	muscle disease or progressive weakness		
23	arthritis		
24	any previous operations – please list i ii iii iv		
25	any anaesthetic or surgical complications – please list i ii iii		

Are you:

		YES	NO
26	pregnant		
27	taking the contraceptive pill		

After your surgery, will you:

		YES	NO
28	be able to be driven home by private car		
29	have someone to take you home		
30	have a telephone at home		
31	have easy access to a lavatory		
32	have someone at home able to look after you for 24 hours		

33 When was your last local or general anaesthetic? ....

34 Has any member of your family had problems with anaesthetic? YES/NO

35 How long will it take you to get home? .... hr ...... mins

36 Do you have any of the following (please circle)

Dentures Crowned teeth Contact lenses Hearing aid Pacemaker

Patient's signature .... Date ....

Assessor ....

Anaesthetist ....

questions may need further explanation. The information provided by the patient and their relatives is then used as a basis for further discussion between the assessing nurse and the patient. The presence of relatives during this discussion should also be actively encouraged; in the case of children, it is clearly essential. Standard screening measures such as height and weight and blood pressure (if appropriate) should be recorded.

Any interview between nurse and patient requires privacy. Ideally, a room with no other purpose should be used, so that patients are not distracted by the presence of equipment or other activity. The interview should have a structured and an unstructured component, both of which require well-developed questioning skills (please see Chapter 4). It is desirable that some consistency is maintained with regard to the provision of pre-operative information, hence the requirement of a structured section. However, it is important that the assessing nurse takes time to find out what patients already know and understand *and starts at that point*. Aspects of physical preparation include the need for fasting and the optimum time and the need for, and extent of, any skin preparation. Procedural information and an outline of the time spent on the unit on the day of surgery may be beneficial to some patients. But, assessing nurses must be able to recognize emotional factors such as fear and anxiety that may prevent patients from assimilating new information, and tailor the discussion accordingly. (More detailed discussion on the recognition and management of anxiety is to be found in Chapter 7.)

The importance of simple, unambiguous written material to back up verbal information is clearly evident. However, any written material must use simple, jargon-free language so that it may still be understood in a different context, when patients return home and review it with friends and family (see Chapter 7).

> Professional language is not well understood by patients. Nurses and others have to learn to use everyday language so that their traditional words are not a barrier to patient involvement. (Wright 1995)

The presence of a supporting relative or friend is also encouraged. Indeed, it could be argued that much of the information regarding discharge and immediate postoperative management is just as appropriate to relatives, if not more so.

For young children, written information might take the form of a story or colouring book that is reviewed with the child and their parents at pre-admission assessment. This time gives day surgery nurses the opportunity to explore the child's previous experience of hospital, any fears or inaccurate beliefs they or the parents may have and the parents' ability to support the child (Burden 1993). Clear factual information regarding transport and discharge requirements should be provided. At a recent day surgery conference, a nurse spoke rather disparagingly of a father who arrived to take his child home after a general anaesthetic *on a motorbike*. But was the child pre-assessed? And if so, was the father present? It is quite possible that the mother accompanied the child to pre-admission assessment and learned that the child had to be taken home by private transport. The motorbike was that transport, and the father duly turned up to collect his child. This example underlines the need for absolute clarity and the involvement where possible, of the carer at pre-admission assessment. We would strongly argue that regardless of the patient's age, pre-admission assessment is for both patient and carer.

The unstructured component of the pre-admission assessment interview will vary in length and content between patients. At the minimum level, nurses must be prepared to ask patients if there is anything at all that they wish to ask about or discuss, and to demonstrate non-verbally that they are genuinely interested in what they have to say. Too often, nurses ask this question on the way out of the door which gives a very clear message to patients. As pointed out by Dutton (1994) the educational, psychological and support needs of some patients go far beyond what is routinely provided at pre-admission assessment; this must be explicitly recognized and catered for.

Summary

> Expansion of day surgery can only safely continue if patients at risk are identified correctly before the procedure. (Irvine *et al.* 1995)

Nurse-led pre-admission assessment based on sound and agreed criteria represents the most logical and ideal means of selecting and preparing patients for a wide range of day surgery procedures. But whilst the screening element of the role attracts the evaluative studies and appears to be taking precedence in the available literature, the educative/support element is essential to the development and maintenance of quality patient care. Nurses have a unique role to play in providing consistency and support in a fast-moving service that often fails to take account fully of the unique needs of the individual. In order for patients to obtain the full benefits of a comprehensive pre-admission assessment programme, nurses need to accept that their role in the process goes far beyond that of taking blood pressures and simple information giving, and that appropriate staff training and development must be a priority for day surgery managers.

Key Points

- Rigorous assessment and screening are the key to continued safe expansion of day surgery services.
- The selection of procedures should be based on the operating time, and current anaesthetic and surgical practice.
- Patients' suitability should be assessed on individual pathology, general medical fitness, their social circumstances and fitness for general anaesthetic.
- Pre-admission assessment comprises two equally important elements; pre-operative screening and education/support.
- Comprehensive and sensitive pre-admission assessment will therefore facilitate thorough appraisal of patient suitability, development of nurse–patient relationships and the provision of support and education. Interviews should have both a structured and unstructured component.
- Pre-admission assessment should be organized in such a way that makes the most efficient use of resources, whilst remaining responsive to patients' needs and should include relatives/carers whenever possible.

Recommended Reading

Markanday, L. and Platzer, H. (1994) **Brief encounters.** *Nursing Times* **90**(7): 38–42

A comprehensive article exploring pre-admission assessment in relation to Orem's model

References

American Society of Anaesthesiology (1991) **ASA classification of surgical patients.** Chicago: ASA.

Audit Commission (1990) **A short cut to better services – Day surgery in England & Wales.** London: HMSO.

Audit Commission (1991) **Measuring quality: The patient's view of day surgery.** London: HMSO.

Bloor, K. and Maynard, A. (1994) **Through the keyhole.** *The Health Service Journal* **104**(5429) 17 Nov: 24–26.

Bottrill, P. (1994) **Nursing assessment prior to day surgery.** *Journal of One-Day Surgery* **4**(2): 22–23.

Bridger, P. and Rees, M. (1995) **What a difference a day makes.** *The Health Service Journal* **105**(5449) 20 April: 22–23.

Burden, N. (1993) **Ambulatory Surgery Nursing.** Philadelphia: Saunders.

Callaghan, L. C., Edwards, N. D. and Reilly, C. S. (1995) **Utilisation of the pre-operative ECG.** *Anaesthesia* **50**: 488–490.

Davies, P. R. F. and Ogg, T. W. (1993) **Managing anaesthesia for geriatric day surgery.** *Journal of One Day Surgery* Spring 93: 16–18.

Dobson, F. (1992) **Health Promotion: a role for peri-operative nurses.** *Journal of Clinical Nursing* **1**: 253–258.

Draper, P. (1987) **Not a job for juniors.** *Nursing Times* **83**(10): 58–62.

Dutton, K. A. (1994) **Patient education in a day surgery unit.** *Journal of One-Day Surgery* **3**(4): 22–24.

Edwards, N. D. and Riley, C. S. (1994) **Detection of perioperative myocardial ischaemia.** *British Journal of Anaesthesia* Vol 72: 104–115.

Ellerton, M. L. and Merriam, C. (1994) **Preparing children and families psychologically for day surgery: an evaluation.** *Journal of Advanced Nursing* **19**: 1057–1062.

Ewles, L. & Simnett, I. (1992) **Promoting Health: A practical guide** (Second Edition). London: Scutari.

Farquharson, M. (1993) **Day surgery for patients over 70 years old.** *Journal of One-day Surgery* (Summer 93): 20–22.

Farrelly, H. and Lakeman, D. (1993) **Patient education in day care.** *Journal of One-Day Surgery* **3**(3): 18–20.

Hatfield, A. and Tronson, M. (1992) **The Complete Recovery Room Book**. New York: Oxford.

Haynes, S. R. and Awler, P. G. T. (1995) **An assessment of the consistency of ASA physical status classification allocation.** *Anaesthesia* **50**: 195–199.

Irvine, C., White, J. and Ingoldby, C. J. (1995) **Nurse screening before intermediate day case surgery.** *Journal of One-Day Surgery* **4**(3): 5–7.

Jarrett, P. (1989) **Operations in day surgery.** In Bradshaw E. G. and Davenport H. T. (Eds) *Day Care: Surgery, Anaesthesia & Management.* London: Edward Arnold.

Markanday, L. and Platzer, H. (1994) **Brief encounters.** *Nursing Times* **90**(7): 38–42.

NHS ME (1993) **Day surgery: Report by the day surgery task force.** Heywood: BAPS Health Publications Unit.

NHS ME Value for Money Unit (1991) **Day surgery – Making it happen.** London: HMSO.

Norris, E. (1992) **Care of the paediatric day surgery patient.** *British Journal of Nursing* **1**(11): 547–551.

RCR Working Party (1989) **Making best use of a department of radiology: Guidelines for doctors.** London: Royal College of Radiologists.

Royal College of Surgeons of England (1992) **Report of the working party on guidelines for day case surgery** (Revised Edition). London: RCoS.

Royle, J. A. and Walsh, M. (1992) **Watson's Medical–Surgical Nursing & Related Physiology** (Fourth Edition). London: Baillière Tindall.

Vijay, V., King, T. A. and Knowles, L. (1995) **Preliminary experience of a day surgery assessment clinic.** *Journal of One-Day Surgery* **4**(3): 7–8.

Wright, S. (1995) **We thought we knew ... Involving patients in nursing practice – an executive summary.** London: Kings Fund & Nursing Development Units.

Chapter 6 Nursing theory and models of care in day surgery

Overview

With the numbers of patients coming through day surgery units increasing and the nature of surgery becoming more complex, it is important that necessary nursing documentation and other paperwork be kept to a minimum. It is essential, therefore, that nurses are able to utilize a framework for assessing and planning care that is quick and simple to use, whilst at the same time, remaining sensitive to individual patient need.

Few nursing models lend themselves exclusively to discrete areas of practice; day surgery requires a flexible approach to care planning and documentation that will meet not only the needs of both adult and child patients but also the demands of a fast-moving service. To take account of these potentially differing needs, the discussion within this chapter actively encourages and promotes the adoption of an eclectic approach to assessing, planning, delivering and evaluating care in day surgery settings. All practitioners must be able to 'own' the model or framework utilized in their area of practice, so this chapter explores critically a couple of the familiar and more commonly used models in order to promote reflection and, hopefully, the development of local initiatives. The increase in use of standard care plans is also discussed in relation to both safety standards and legal requirements.

Chapter Focus

- The nursing process and nursing models
- The concept of self-care
- Nursing models used in day surgery settings
- Standard care plans and legal aspects of record keeping
- Assessment and care planning
- Collaborative care

Introduction

The day of surgery is usually considered to be a particularly anxious time both for patients and their carers; the importance of a warm and welcoming initial reception cannot be overemphasized. In addition, an admission procedure that is simple, quick and safe whilst taking account of individual concerns can do much to reduce this anxiety. Patients undergoing day surgery vary considerably in age, expectations and experiences, but nurses working in the specialty, whilst striving to provide individualized care, often find themselves hamstrung by rigid and confining examples of nursing documentation. These in reality are often little more than checklists that in themselves promote automatic and non-critical performance and offer few opportunities for deviation and attention to the differing needs of patients.

Truly individualized care needs a more flexible approach to documentation, that is based on a more logical way of *thinking* about nursing care. The shortness of stay characteristic of day surgery does not exempt nurses from this way of thinking; so let us return to the nursing process.

The Nursing Process and Nursing Models

Up until the late 1960s many nurses believed that good nursing practice was founded on instinct and empathy, an approach now challenged for its reliance on intuition at the expense of rational thought. Yura and Walsh (1967) were amongst the first to call for a more systematic assessment of patients' needs, going on to identify the now familiar stages of the process of nursing:

- assessment
- planning
- implementation
- evaluation.

For the first time nurses were being actively encouraged to monitor and appraise the effectiveness of the care they were giving. Despite its many criticisms, the process seeks to involve the patient or client in decisions about care, and any system that achieves this goal represents a considerable move forward. However, its introduction in this country is testament to the lack of clarity and real understanding surrounding the nursing process and the role of models within the profession as a whole (de la Cuesta 1983). The expression *nursing process* has also been subject to question; Walsh and Ford (1989) suggest it be replaced by the term 'individualized patient care', as this is clearer and more accurate. The nursing process was never conceived as a model in itself, rather more as a logical way of thinking; a recognition that nursing is a process, not a set of unrelated activities. This process is graphically represented as a simple and effective four-stage problem-solving cycle (Fig. 6.1). It is the tool with which to put a nursing

Figure 6.1 The problem-solving cycle of the nursing process

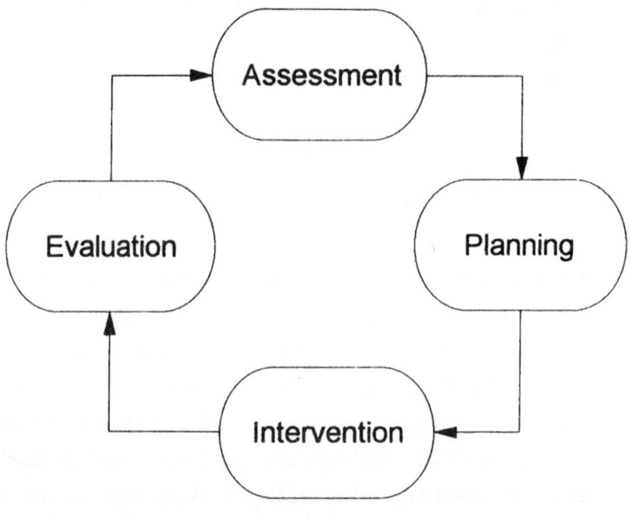

model into practice. The nursing process aims to promote more systematic and rationally planned nursing care, and to reduce the more ritualistic and haphazard aspects of practice.

Nursing Models

Most nurses have, at some time during their practice been required to come to terms with a nursing model, usually under duress and often with extremely limited motivation; again, the term itself can be off-putting. Although they seem quite abstract, they do in fact provide a means of understanding and explaining the things that nurses actually do. Riehl and Roy (1980) offer this definition of a nursing model:

> . . . a systematically constructed, scientifically based and logically related set of concepts which identify the essential components of nursing practice, together with the theoretical basis of these concepts and values required for their use by the practitioner . . .

– quite a complex definition for a complex concept. A more simple definition put forward by Dylak (1986) identifies a model as 'a comprehensive definition of the roles and functions of the nurse'. This latter definition places rightful emphasis on nursing *roles* and *behaviours* which form the core of all nursing frameworks or models. But however defined, nursing models are not simply a few random opinions of out of touch and mostly American nurse theorists who have not seen or touched a patient for years (as their critics appear to believe). They are developed logically in order that nurses may think more logically about the things they do. The major problem with the more formal models is that the language used is often unfamiliar and complicated, which tends to obscure essential meanings and certainly does not make for easy reading.

But when defined in more simple terms, it does become easy to appreciate that most nurses carry their own model for practice, whether or not they are aware of it. Robinson (1990) calls these 'occupational theories', usually representing common-sense ideas that help nurses do the job they are involved with and are developed from experience. Sometimes they relate closely to other occupations. For example, some nurses value foremost the carrying out of doctors' orders in the most efficient manner. The patient is a recipient of care that is largely derived from medical prescription; loosely this can be referred to as a *medical model of care.* Whilst there is nothing wrong with this in itself, and there are many occasions when patients need and want just this sort of approach, it is perhaps rather narrow to cast *all* patients in this somewhat passive role.

Other nurses actively encourage patients and clients to evaluate their own health status and assist them to identify potential and actual problems, related to daily living activities or health needs, and thereby promoting self-care and independence. The patient's role is different here, more of a partner in the provision of care and the model loosely defined as self-care. Again, it would be wrong to assume that all patients want, or indeed are able, to take such an active role in their care.

The differences between these two approaches begs the question of what precisely a nursing model should be concerned with. Clearly, they should be developed in order to improve nursing practice; unfortunately, the implicit message is that present practice is flawed and inadequate and therefore models have largely been greeted with hostility and suspicion. According to Aggleton and Chalmers (1986) a nursing model should address the following:

- the nature of people
- the causes of problems likely to require nursing intervention
- the nature of the assessment process
- the nature of the planning and goal-setting process
- the focus of intervention during the implementation of the care plan
- the nature of the process of evaluating the quality and effects of the care given
- the role of the nurse.

This list is particularly helpful, not only in assisting in evaluation of published nursing models, but also as a means of developing new frameworks. For example, what can you say about the nature of people who are in your care? First, that they are whole *people*, not just patients, they are of different ages and backgrounds, they are mothers or fathers, husbands or wives, part of a family, etc.

The activities model and the self-care model, whilst obviously not the only two approaches to care management available, probably underpin most of the care given in general acute ward settings. The self-care model, frequently referred to in day surgery contexts, is explored below.

Self-care and Autonomy in the Context of Day Surgery

The term 'self-care' is somewhat ambiguous. Frequently, nurses have defined their patients as 'self-caring' largely when they are not requiring any specific nursing intervention other than administering medication or changing a dressing. In this context, the term seems to imply that the patient is independently meeting their own needs, and is what most plans of care document as their outcomes. In other words, the patient has returned to carrying out those activities of life that they would normally do without conscious thought. Schober (1989) believes that this actually means that the patient is receiving no care, and argues that this idea of 'DIY' care needs to be challenged.

However, another more specific use of the term self-care is to be found within Dorothea Orem's self-care model for nursing (Orem 1991). The model, first published in 1971, encompasses three major constructs:

- self-care
- self-care deficit
- nursing.

Orem defines self-care as 'the practice of activities that individuals initiate and perform on their own behalf in maintaining life, health and well-being'; these are learned behaviours, shaped and influenced by social and cultural factors, and directed towards meeting *universal, developmental* and *health deviation* needs. According to Orem, people are functional wholes, capable of predetermined action and are motivated to achieve self-care; that is, to maintain a sense of balance. She therefore sees self-care as a purposeful action and also by definition, beneficial to people's health. Health is defined by Orem as a state of 'soundness or wholeness of developed human structures and of bodily and mental functioning' – not the clearest of definitions.

The *universal* needs are applicable to everyone and are concerned with normal functioning, both in physical and psycho-social terms. They are:

- sufficient intake of air, water and food
- maintenance of elimination
- balance between activity and rest
- balance between social interaction and solitude
- prevention of hazards
- promotion of development and potential.

Developmental needs are more life-stage specific and relate to events which may affect self-care ability, and would include, for example, marriage, childbirth, redundancy or divorce. Together, universal and developmental needs represent the nature of self-care in relation to health maintenance and promotion.

Orem assumes that a 'healthy' person has sufficient self-care abilities to meet these needs. But when the person has to cope with illness, they are likely to have additional demands; that is, *health deviation* needs. Orem also refers to this as *therapeutic self-care demand*, and it is affected by a number of conditioning factors, including socio-cultural and environmental factors as well as past experiences.

The usefulness of the model in explaining differences in response to illness lies in its accord with those previously discussed in relation to lay interpretations of illness and illness behaviour (see Chapter 3). The relationship between these factors and health is therefore implicit within the model, but it is important to acknowledge that whilst individuals seek to maintain control over their lives in general, and perhaps as we have seen, their *health*, they do not necessarily wish to retain that level of autonomy in decisions about the management of specific *disease*. Orem, however, postulates that when the individual is able to meet the additional demands of illness from their existing abilities, balance is therefore maintained and intervention is not required. This clearly concurs with available evidence on the extent of self-care within the community (Scambler 1991). *Nursing*, as defined by Orem, is only required when a deficit exists between self-care ability (of the individual and others) and their self-care demand, and it is precisely upon this premise that most day surgery units using the model have justified their selection. To what extent the model really addresses the needs of all patient groups within the speciality is open to question; clearly, a major factor in such a discussion concerns patients expectations, both of the efficacy of the proposed treatment options, their care whilst in hospital and their subsequent recovery. According to Orem, there are three nursing systems:

- *Wholly compensatory*; that is, the patient has no active role in their care; the nurse does for and acts for the patient. In the context of day surgery, this would correspond to the period when the patient is anaesthetized.
- *Partly compensatory*; that is, nurse and patient share in the performance of care, which will vary according to the patient's knowledge and abilities. This type of nursing intervention relates to the roles in immediate pre- and postoperative care.
- *Educative/supportive*; that is, the teaching and support of patients in the performance of their own care. This aspect of nursing function could relate to pre-admission assessment, pre-discharge planning and postoperative management at home.

Intervention and assistance may be provided by nurses, other members of the care team, family members or friends and may involve:

- doing or acting for another (includes the advocate role)
- guiding and directing for another (providing information and/or advice)
- providing physical support (a partnership)
- providing psychological support (empathic presence)
- providing an environment which supports development
- teaching another.

Cavanagh (1991) points out that these actions are not mutually exclusive, and there are plenty of occasions when different types of nursing intervention are carried out at the same time. For example, during a pre-admission assessment interview, the nurse will be teaching providing information which is clearly based on both physical and psychological support. Similarly, the giving of immediate postoperative care, is likely to be accompanied by discussion and education in relation to discharge and subsequent care at home.

Much of the criticism surrounding Orem's model lies in its rather obscure terminology; the use of terms such as 'technologic-professional operations' (essentially her term for the nursing process) do little for the reader trying to get to grips with the major concepts. This is not just a question of semantics; the lack of operational clarity renders such constructs unquantifiable, and difficult to evaluate. As Cavanagh (1991) asks, 'If nurses are not completely clear about the meaning, application and recording of the model's tenets, how is consistency in practice to develop?'. That said, there is nothing to stop nurses defining the constructs within the context of their own practice and adopting a more workable terminology to accompany them. Nursing models are not absolutes; like nurses themselves, they need to grow and adapt to changing circumstances and needs.

Another source of contention lies with Orem's quite fixed belief that people want to be self-caring and that this is a quite deliberate activity; there is little evidence to suggest that this is always the case, and indeed there are plenty of examples around that suggest otherwise.

But at face value, the relevance of Orem's model to day surgery practice seems clear. The basic philosophy of self-care seems to fit with an area of nursing where most of the pre-operative and postoperative care is carried out by the patients themselves at home with help from family and friends. The explicit teaching, advocacy and support roles of the nurse are likewise relevant and Orem's assertion that it is up to individual nurses to apply the model in practice do indeed make it a logical choice for day surgery settings. It is a pity that there are no published, more comprehensive accounts of the model in practice; greater clarity and simplification of terms and worked examples would do much to encourage others to adopt the basic concepts as a framework for all nursing care from pre-admission assessment to discharge. Some accounts of the model's use refer only to the adoption of universal self-care requisites as a check list for assessment; rarely are the different categories of nursing action described by the model fully outlined and evaluated. However, this does not apply to day surgery; in practice the use of models, formal or otherwise often appears to stop at the assessment stage.

As we have seen previously, the concept of self-care underpins much that is written on health behaviour (see Chapter 3). Health education and health promotion are being increasingly acknowledged as fundamental aspects of the nurse's role in acute care settings, although it is not always easy to identify specific instances where such intervention may be appropriate.

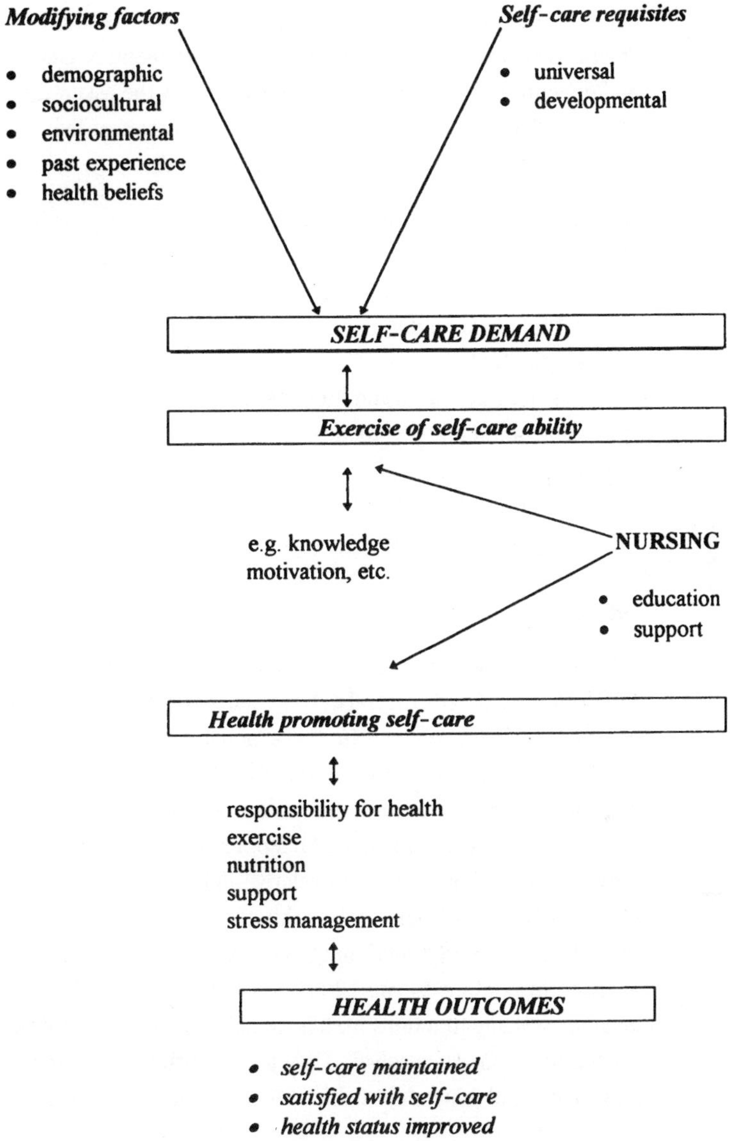

Figure 6.2 Relationships between self-care and health protection (adapted from Simmons 1990)

Simmons (1990) offers a framework to help identify the relationships between factors that may influence people's ability to make healthy choices and protect their health. She uses Orem's concept of self-care as a basis for explaining ideas about specific health-promoting behaviours that people are believed to undertake. The framework (see Fig. 6.2) may prove useful for day surgery nurses as a broad guide to thinking about and planning health-promotion approaches, though it appears to suffer from the same lack of evaluation and reliability as the health belief model outlined in Chapter 3.

Life as Activities

The activities model is probably the one most familiar to nurses in the UK. Nancy Roper and her colleagues sought to identify key qualities common to all human beings, and in doing so, they chose to focus on activities people perform, rather than on needs. Activities were thought more amenable to observation and therefore measurement. Needs, on the other hand, are more abstract and difficult to quantify. The model is based on the assumption that people are best understood by the activities they perform. The list of activities of living (ALs) was eventually revised to 12 from 16 and these are said to be *related* to needs:

- maintaining a safe environment
- communicating
- breathing
- eating and drinking
- eliminating
- personal cleansing and dressing
- controlling body temperature
- mobilizing
- working and playing
- expressing sexuality
- sleeping
- dying.

As you can see, most of these activities are physiologically determined, though some have rather thinly defined cultural determinants. Roper *et al.* (1983) argue that people can and do vary considerably with respect to these activities; factors such as age, past experience, choice, education and opportunity will clearly influence both the degree of independence and ability. The causes of problems for individuals move them from a state of relative independence to one of relative dependence for a given AL. For example, the administration of a general anaesthetic will move a person from a state of relative independence to one of absolute dependence for most essential activities such as breathing, maintaining a safe environment, and mobilizing. An individual's *normal* functioning (i.e. in health) and present functioning (i.e. in illness) are assessed in relation to the 12 activities. According to Roper *et al.*, the nursing role may then encompass many functions from information giving to carrying out, in total, ALs that patients are unable to do for themselves. They also identify three further nursing behaviours: preventing, comforting and dependent behaviour. These are directed towards:

- maintaining health
- promoting independence
- preventing ill-health and injury
- enhancing self-care

– according to the individual's capacity.

How each activity is carried out, how often, where and when will vary according to their stage in the lifespan. According to Roper *et al.*, the individual's main objective in carrying out these activities is to attain self-fulfilment and maximum independence within their own limitations. They do not actually define health within the model, rather it is implicit in this defined state of self-fulfilment and independence as judged by the individual. But suppose that an individual patient does not want to be self-fulfilled and independent; is he or she unhealthy? Does a nurse have the right to try and alter the patient's view? If the individual patient does not think that he or she has a problem, what should the nurse do? These are important questions to ask.

Much of the criticism levelled at the activities model stems from its theoretical base which does not appear to be adequately justified; there is no evidence to suggest that all human beings seek self-fulfilment. Part of this difficulty derives from the authors' acceptance of Maslow's (1970) hierarchy of needs. This hierarchy in itself can be questioned, as needs are not necessarily hierarchical. More importantly, as Webb (1984) points out, Maslow's somewhat sexist and elitist concept of *self-actualization* was only ever meant to apply to a small minority of the population – mostly high achieving *men*, not everyone as Roper and her colleagues suggest. Maslow's ideas are just that; his own ideas about life – they are not based on any empirical evidence.

Walsh (1991), among others, criticizes the model for its rather reductionist approach to the complexity of human life. It relies heavily on the biological sciences, but lacks a psychological or socio-cultural dimension. Walsh rightly asks for the evidence that the 12 activities 'represent a comprehensive and definitive view of human behaviour', and goes on to outline a number of important factors such as self-concept and self-worth, attitudes and beliefs, that are not recognized by the model.

Problems reported with the model in practice are also associated with the 12 activities. Confusion often occurs during assessment because it is not always clear where certain items should be entered. A classic example in a day surgery context would be anxiety that is affecting sleep, appetite and ability to concentrate. This could be placed under communicating; sleeping; eating and drinking; maintaining a safe environment; and working and playing. Other relevant examples are haemorrhage and pain. The activity of expressing sexuality is also contentious; gender expression is probably more accurate. Its popularity appears to lie solely on its almost

Reflection Points

Note down the characteristics of the patient population on your unit. You may need to consider:

- age
- gender
- socio-cultural group
- ethnic group
- first time or repeat attenders
- length of stay on unit
- complexity of procedures.

There will be probably both considerable variation *and* many common characteristics.

- Can one approach to assessment and care planning really meet these potentially different needs?
- What have the two models discussed to offer nursing practice in your unit?
- Where are the shortfalls?
- Can aspects of other models or frameworks help?

checklist format that is written in uncomplicated (except for the sexuality) language. Overall, the model does not appear to have as much to offer day surgery practice as that of Orem.

It is important that a model is evaluated in the context of individual areas of practice. What appears to work on one unit need not necessarily work on another; it may be worthwhile trying to identify the factors within your unit that mitigate against the use of a given model or framework.

A major illustrative example is provided by children in a day surgery context. The approach to assessment and care and the role of the nurse must explicitly take the needs and expectations of parents into account. Casey's model (1988) is based on the concept of partnership:

> The care of children, well or sick, is best carried out by their families, with varying degrees of assistance from members of a suitably qualified health care team whenever necessary. (Casey 1988)

The model distinguishes between family care (care of the child, given by the child or family) and nursing care, which should only be given when family resources are insufficient for that particular instance. Casey does not advocate fixed boundaries between these two constructs, but promotes partnership between the family and nursing staff. Consequently, *family care* may be given by the nurse if the family is unable or absent and *nursing care* can be given by the family with appropriate teaching and support. Essential elements therefore within Casey's model to the building of a sense of partnership are the teaching, support and referral roles of the nurse. These roles are not dissimilar to those advocated by Orem, and once more appear to describe the varied role of the nurse in day surgery.

No one model can be used exclusively; adopting an eclectic approach has many advantages and is probably the way to proceed. The language used within the framework is important and needs to be understandable but even more important is the *meaning*; there must be a common understanding. According to Pearson and Vaughan (1986), if a nursing team can agree on a framework, be it a formal model or otherwise, some possible advantages can be identified:

- greater consistency of care received by patients
- improved direction to nursing care; goals and outcomes are understood by all
- provides a guide to decision and policy-making
- helps to guide the criteria by which new staff are selected.

Assessment

Assessment, as Walsh (1991) suggests, is the most important stage in individualized patient care; without it he believes that 'all patients are treated much the same with only their medical diagnosis having any influence on care'. The term covers a number of activities, including the collection and review of information and the identification of actual and potential problems; the essential components are an assessment tool and an assessing nurse. Just as nursing care is only as good as the information upon which it is based, so is the assessment format is only as good as the skills of the nurse who completes it. Those required for assessment are:

- observation skills
- interviewing skills
- measurement skills

– within a framework that is realistic and suitable for day surgery patients. Professional judgement and discussion between the nursing team is needed in deciding just what is and what is not necessary. Walsh and Ford (1989) argue that a common complaint about the use of the nursing process is that the paperwork is cumbersome, but relatively few nurses have set about personalizing their nursing assessment format in a rational and systematic way.

In the context of day surgery, much of the initial nursing assessment will have been completed at pre-admission assessment interview, assuming of course that all patients are pre-assessed. Once again, we emphasize the importance of ensuring that all pre-admission assessments take place no more than 4–6 weeks before the proposed date of surgery.

Necessary questions relating to general medical, social and anaesthetic fitness can either be incorporated into a nursing assessment form based on the chosen model or framework, or remain as a separate questionnaire. There are probably benefits and limitations attached to each option. If the integrated option is chosen, a level of compromise may be necessary to ensure clarity with respect to judgements about suitability, whilst trying to avoid the use of endless tick-box forms that offer little scope for expansion and recording of individual concerns.

According to Aggleton and Chalmers (1986), assessment that is based on Orem's model first seeks to determine whether there is a deficit (problem) arising between self-care ability (what the patient can do) and self-care demand (what the patient is being asked to do both pre- and postoperatively). Second, assessment seeks to determine whether that deficit (problem) is due to lack of knowledge, skill or motivation or some past experience; in the context of day surgery, problems are largely due to past experience, and/or lack of knowledge or skill.

Planning

Any problems identified during either pre-admission or admission interview should be documented, appropriate goals set and ways of achieving these goals discussed with the patient. In reality, these stages tend to proceed concurrently as much of the nursing role is concerned with teaching and support of patients. However, it is still essential that identified problems and goals are documented and there are different ways of achieving this. One method is that of a common core plan. Some examples of standard plans (pre-operative and postoperative care) are outlined in Chapters 7 and 11.

Standardized Care Plans – Standardized Care or Setting Standards for Quality?

Over a period of time in a day surgery unit it is likely that a large number of patients will present with similar problems. These may include lack of knowledge and experience of the effects of general anaesthetic, fears about possible effects of general anaesthetic (e.g. feeling, and being, sick), anxiety about possible problems at home, etc. These are essentially problems common to many surgical patients, and as such are frequently documented in *common core* care plans. A central concern in day surgery is the provision and maintenance of quality care and services. A more comprehensive discussion relating to quality, standards and monitoring is to be found in Chapter 12, but it is useful to consider the issue of standards here as well. In areas of good practice, common care plans provide the basis for the setting of objectives and quality standards to improve patient outcomes. An outcome is defined by Donabedian (1980) as 'a change in the patient's current and future health (including psychological and social health) and behaviour that can be attributed to antecedent care'. If care plans are written as specific and measurable standards then audit processes may assess the contribution of nursing intervention in achieving improved patient outcomes; according to Snowley *et al.* (1992), standard-setting represents the first step in the audit cycle. The following categories of measurable outcomes are adapted from Millar (1993):

- patient satisfaction
- patient knowledge or understanding of their illness
- functional health status
- clinical health status
- psychosocial health status
- patient's disposition
- complications (e.g. infection rates)
- discharge
- patient compliance.

Do care plans reflect these outcomes? The question to be answered here is to what extent nurses recognize that assessment and care planning are essential elements of what Donabedian terms 'antecedent care'. The fact is that care planning and care giving are inextricably linked; writing care plans must not be seen as a irritating distraction from 'real' nursing. In statutory terms they are one and the same. These are important issues and worth considering when attempting to develop core plans as a time-saving exercise.

Whilst the advantages of core plans are measurable in terms of time saved recording information (Walsh 1991) it is, however, vital that aspects of individuality are not lost in the process; patient assessment must always be carried out and nursing documentation must allow for integration of individual problems. The use of this type of care plan in day surgery appears to be a logical solution to documentation in a fast-moving service, but some caution and a clear understanding of their use are required. There is a world of difference between systematically defining problems that are common to patients undergoing day surgery procedures and simply assuming that all patients are the same, and by definition, require the same care. The latter view equates the common-core care plan with routinized and often minimal care and that is exactly what must be avoided.

Conversely, there is no gain in having a core care plan that lists dozens of potential problems that will rarely materialize; the approach adopted should be a rational one, but one that addresses the total peri-operative period. For example, problems common to patients pre-operatively might include lack of knowledge and anxiety. (That the patient needs to be prepared for surgery is a nursing requirement or problem, not a patient problem – this frequently causes difficulty on care plans.) Other problems are identified for the intra-operative period and first- and second-stage recovery. They should document relevant safety information and be signed by the named or primary nurse. As previously mentioned, there must be room on the care plan for recording of specific individual problems or concerns; perhaps more importantly, day surgery nurses need to recognize *explicitly* that people are individual, they will respond to surgery in different ways and will often require more than the 'usual' care.

Legal Aspects of Record Keeping

Nurses frequently appear confused as to what does and what does not constitute a legal document. The answer is that anything that the court chooses to see becomes a legal document (Dimond 1995). This point is also made by the United Kingdom Central Council for Nursing, Midwifery and Health Visiting (UKCC); 'Any document which records any aspect of the care of a patient or client can be required as evidence before a court of law …' (UKCC 1993). It is perhaps worthwhile to return to the rationale for creating and keeping records in order that their importance can be seen in context. The paper *Standards for Records and Record Keeping,* published by the UKCC (1993) was distributed to all nurses, midwives and health visitors on the professional register; early reading or rereading is recommended. It lays out the following reasons for keeping records. They provide:

- full information concerning patient or client condition and care
- a record of problems arising and any actions taken
- evidence of care required, intervention and patient or client response
- a record of physical, psychological or social factors affecting the patient or client
- a record of events and decision-making
- a baseline record against which to judge improvement or deterioration.

The UKCC add that properly maintained nursing and other records will help patients to become more involved in their care, but only when written in terms they can understand. Records can also help to identify factors that place patients at risk, and help protect nursing staff against any future complaint made. Clear, legible, unambiguous and indelible writing is therefore essential. Each record should be dated and signed, and alterations if necessary made by crossing out with a single line; the bottom line is that the nursing record 'demonstrates that the practitioner's duty of care has been fulfilled' (UKCC 1993). In addition to nursing care plans, operating lists and registers, drug registers, accident forms and recovery sheets are defined as records and governed by the same principles; all are in everyday use in day surgery units. Wicker (1990) offers the following further pointers to good report writing which would be acceptable in court:

- Abbreviations are hazardous because of the likelihood of misinterpretation; therefore they should be avoided.
- Reports should be factual and concise.
- False statements made about patients' risk liability for character defamation.
- Humorous entries in care plans may become defamatory when read out in court.
- Carelessly written reports may leave nurses open to action for negligence.

Recent developments in 'shared care' or collaborative care planning promote interaction between different groups of health professionals and a multidisciplinary approach to care planning and intervention. Each multidisciplinary team (MDT) member is responsible for making entries within a single record. Lancaster (1993) defines collaborative care planning (CCP) as 'an explicit multi-disciplinary statement of roles and responsibilities in the field of patient care' and can be developed to include all aspects of a care episode from pre-admission assessment, through day of surgery and back to the community. Lancaster identifies the stages of collaborative care planning (Fig. 6.3).

Figure 6.3 Collaborative care planning

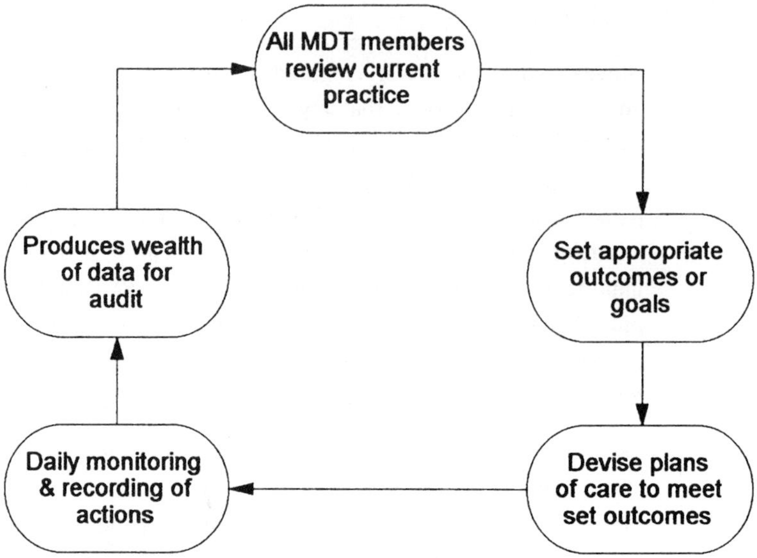

The purpose of collaborative care planning is to ensure that resources are used effectively and that quality of care is defined, monitored and audited. A number of benefits can be realized from adopting a collaborative approach to care planning and documentation. These include benefits to patients through improved information exchange and access to records and to staff through improved communication and understanding of team members' contribution to the care process. However, this again underlines the requirement for accurate record-keeping.

There are doubtless a number of core nursing care plans that would not bear too close scrutiny in legal terms. Just because the care plan is pre-written, does not mean that the nurses' responsibility towards documentation is in some way absolved. In this instance, nurses must accept responsibility for signing up to a care plan that possibly fails to reflect the needs or problems of patients in their care; the full implications of being the 'named nurse' are worthy of individual consideration. When time is short and pressures mount, how easy is it to either sign just the core plan, or worse still, not sign it at all?

Summary

The need for straightforward and realistic nursing documentation in day surgery is clear. But given the potential variation in patient experience, expectation and needs, nurses must utilize or develop a framework or model that facilitates assessment, planning, implementation and evaluation of nursing care. The basic philosophy and roles described in Orem's self-care model appears to reflect much of what day surgery nurses are trying to achieve, but no one model will adequately meet the needs of all patients in all units. Critical evaluation of existing models and the adoption of an eclectic approach to framework development is therefore recommended.

Whilst the common core plan also has much to offer the nurse in day surgery, it needs to be used with caution, and the need for accurate record-keeping made a priority. But there must always be room for identification of individual concerns and nurses must be prepared to ask the right questions to realize the answers. Good common core plans can provide baseline objectives for the setting of quality standards and with the advent of collaborative care planning, the opportunity for multidisciplinary audit.

Key Points

- As numbers of patients undergoing day surgery increase, so does the need for a rational yet sensitive approach to documenting nursing action.
- The shortness of patients stay does not preclude them from comprehensive assessment and planning of care.
- In order for consistency, assessment and planning should be based on a commonly understood framework.
- Formal nursing models need to be evaluated critically in the context of day surgery, adapted accordingly and adopt a more 'user-friendly' language.
- Of the published models, that of Orem (1991) appears to offer the most for day surgery nursing.
- Assessment and care planning must be seen as integral aspects of nursing in day surgery, not unwelcome distractions.
- Core plans can save time and provide the opportunity for setting standards for both nursing practice and nursing care; in practice this is often not the case.
- Regardless of how nursing care is documented, nurses have a statutory responsibility to maintain signed, accurate records of their actions.

Recommended Reading

Cavanagh, S. J. (1991) **Orem's Model in Action.** London: Macmillan

Clear and balanced review of Orem's model. For those who are interested, there is a whole series looking at the more popular models

References

Aggleton, P. and Chalmers, H. (1986) **Nursing Models & the Nursing Process.** London: Macmillan.

Casey, A. (1988) **A partnership with child and family.** *Senior Nurse* **8**(4): 8–9.

Cavanagh, S. J. (1991) **Orem's Model in Action.** London: Macmillan.

De la Cuesta, C. (1983) **The nursing process: from development to implementation.** *Journal Of Advanced Nursing* **8**: 365–371.

Dimond, B. (1995) **Legal Aspects of Nursing** (Second Edition). London: Prentice Hall.

Donabedian, A. (1980) **The Definition of Quality Assurance and Approaches to its Measurement.** Ann Arbor: Health Administration Press.

Dylak, P. (1986) **The State of the Art?** *Nursing Times* **82**(32): 72.

Lancaster, M. (1993) **Collaborative care planning – an orthopaedic experience in Solihull.** *Surgical Nurse* **6**(5): 20–26.

Maslow, A. (1970) **Motivation and Personality** (Second Edition). New York: Harper & Row.

Millar, B. (1993) **The nursing outcomes dilemma.** *Surgical Nurse* **6**(1): 25–29.

Orem, D. E. (1991) **Nursing: Concepts of practice** (Fourth Edition). New York: McGraw-Hill.

Pearson, A. and Vaughan, B. (1986) **Nursing Models for Practice**. London: Heinemann.

Riehl, J. P. and Roy, C. (Eds) (1980) **Conceptual Models for Nursing Practice.** Norwalk, CT: Appleton Century Crofts.

Robinson, K. (1990) **Nursing models – the hidden costs.** *Surgical Nurse* **3**(3): 11–14.

Roper, N., Logan, W. W. and Tierney, A. (1983) **Using a Model for Nursing.** Edinburgh: Churchill Livingstone.

Scambler, G. (Ed.) (1991) **Sociology as Applied to Medicine** (Third Edition). London: Baillière Tindall.

Schober, J. E. (1989) **Approaches to Nursing Care.** In Hinchliff, S. M., Norman, S. E. and Schober, J. E. (Eds) *Nursing Practice & Health Care.* London: Edward Arnold.

Simmons, S. J. (1990) **The health-promoting self-care system model: directions for nursing research and practice.** *Journal of Advanced Nursing* **15**: 1162–1166.

Snowley, G. D., Nicklin, P. J. and Birch, J. A. (1992) **Objectives for Care – Specifying standards for clinical nursing** (Second Edition). London: Wolfe.

UKCC (1993) **Standards for records & record keeping.** London: UKCC.

Walsh, M. (1991) **Models in Clinical Nursing – The way forward.** London: Baillière Tindall.

Walsh, M. and Ford P. (1989) **Nursing Rituals: Research and rational actions.** Oxford: Butterworth–Heinemann.

Webb, C. (1984) **On the eighth day God created the nursing process – and nobody rested!** *Senior Nurse* **1**(33): 22–25.

Wicker, C. P. (1990) **Legal responsibilities of the nurse 1: Introduction to law.** *Surgical Nurse* **3**(5): 12–13.

Yura, H. and Walsh, M. B. (1967) **The Nursing Process.** Norwalk, CT: Appleton Century Crofts.

Chapter 7 Preparation and support of patients prior to anaesthesia

Overview

The prospect of an anaesthetic is often as a great a source of anxiety for people as the operation itself. However, the elimination of that anxiety might not always be in the best interests of patients. '. . . moderate levels of pre-operative anxiety can help patients to prepare for surgery and reduce its stressfulness' (Salmon 1993). This chapter explores some of the theories and manifestations of anxiety, and its effects upon information retention, recall and recovery. In addition, we review some strategies for anxiety management for patients and their carers, in order that more effective support can be provided for patients in the period prior to induction of anaesthesia.

Most of the safety protocols underpinning physical pre-operative preparation are based upon the known effects of general and local anaesthesia. Evaluating current research, this chapter addresses pertinent areas of physical pre-operative preparation.

Chapter Focus

- Theories of anxiety and coping
- Manifestations of anxiety
- Nursing strategies for anxiety reduction
- Means of providing patient support
- Practices in preoperative preparation
- Safety protocols

Introduction

Given that the most commonly identified 'stressors' associated with hospitalization are fear of the unknown, loss of dignity, lack of privacy and loss of control over events, it is not difficult to understand why so many people coming for surgery are anxious. There is now a considerable body of evidence that supports the theory that receiving pre-operative information helps patients prepare for the experience, whilst promoting a greater sense of well-being and a less problematic recovery (e.g. Hayward 1975, Boore 1978, Wilson-Barnett 1980, Hathaway 1986). However, there is also significant evidence which indicates that patients largely fail to communicate their anxieties to nursing staff for a variety of reasons (e.g. Johnson 1980, 1982). As Johnson (1982) points out, if nurses and doctors do not know what worries a patient has, then they are unlikely to be in a position to offer *appropriate* support and reduce the ill effects of *high* levels of anxiety. Furthermore, Markland and Hardy (1993) suggest that individuals having day surgery are amongst the most anxious of all surgical patients. Yet on the day of their operation, patients scheduled for day surgery often need to be admitted and processed quite rapidly, which can result in scant regard for individual fears and concerns. This ongoing scenario gives rise to some important considerations. In the first instance, day surgery nurses need to be more alert to the many different manifestations of anxiety and its effects on the patients in their care. Second, they need to consider the factors, both in their own individual practice and within the unit's environment, which may prevent patients from disclosing their fears.

Theories of Anxiety

Are Stress and Anxiety One and the Same?

It is probably true to say that anxiety is easier to define by its possible manifestations than its possible causes; most of us are able recognize when we feel anxious, but often are unable to explain *why* we feel that way. It is quite common to find the terms *stress* and *anxiety* being used interchangeably. Some theorists underline the importance of separating these two concepts.

Stress

According to Bond (1986) stress can be defined in three major ways:

As a Stimulus

When stress is described in terms of a stimulus there are clearly a large number of potential stressors in our environment: hunger, cold, pain, meeting new people, to name but a few. The limitation of this explanation is that few of these stressors would reliably cause 'stress' in everybody and even if they did, the effects would never be consistent.

As a Response

The idea of stress defined as a response to a stimulus is generally attributed to Hans Selye (1976). His theory holds that the 'stressor' disturbs the body's equilibrium (homoeostasis) and responses mediated by the nervous and endocrine systems' attempt to restore the balance (Fig. 7.1). Termed the General Adaptation Syndrome by Selye, he argued the same processes and systems are involved regardless of the *type* of stressor.

This neuro-endocrine response to stress is essentially a protective and adaptive mechanism with three distinct phases:

- *alarm* – generally attributed to adrenaline and noradrenaline release
- *adaptation (or resistance)* – characterized by circulating glucocorticoids
- *exhaustion* – individual no longer able to respond to stress.

Clearly, prolonged exposure to stressors can have serious implications for health. However, the major limitation of this explanation of stress is that it fails to recognize the importance of psychological mediation in both stimulus (cause) and response (effect).

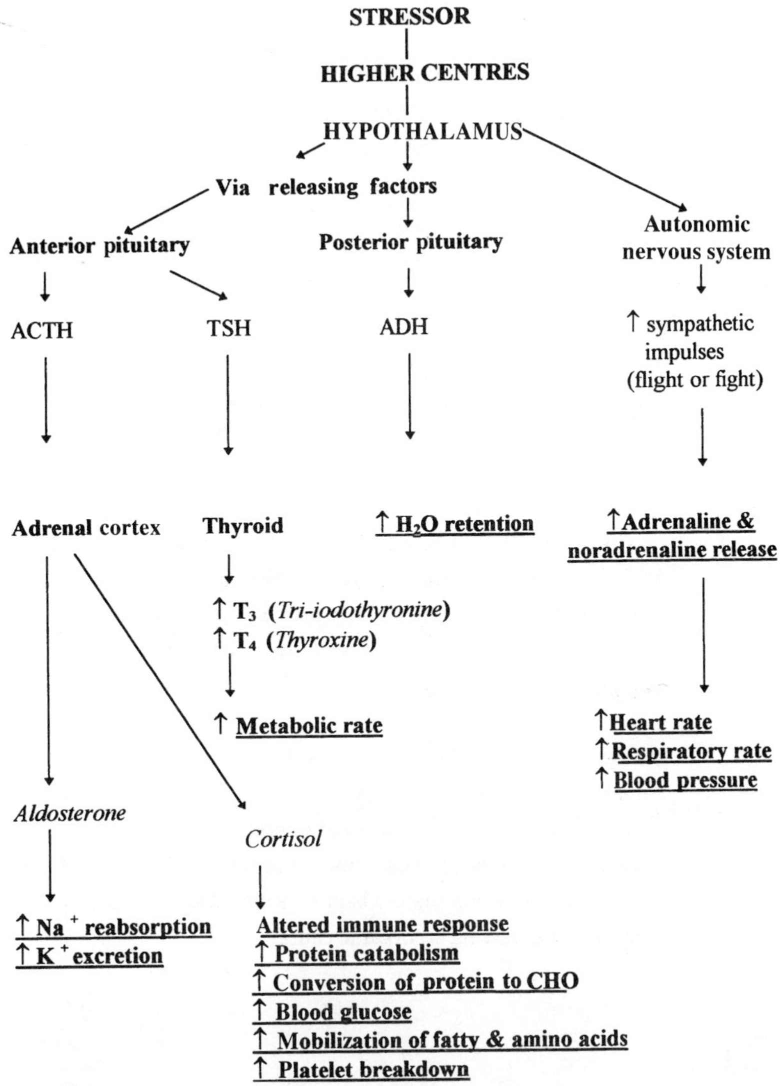

Figure 7.1 Neuroendocrine response to a stressor. ADH, antidiuretic hormone; ACTH, adrenocorticotrophic hormone; TSH, thyroid stimulating hormone; CHO, carbohydrate

As a Transaction

This current view takes the vital cognitive aspect into account and builds on Selye's work. The theory differentiates between *demand* (i.e. the stimulus perceived by the individual as needing a response) and *coping* (i.e. the response that is carried out by the individual and assessed as to its effectiveness). Lazarus (1976) argues that stress is not a quality in an object or situation, rather it is derived from *our interpretation of that situation* or object. To deal with this stress, we have *coping* mechanisms. Coping involves two separate processes: primary and secondary appraisal. Primary appraisal deals with the question, what is the nature of the danger of this situation? Secondary appraisal helps us decide what can be done about the situation. Stress is said to arise from the individual's appraisal of a mismatch between the demand placed upon them and their ability to cope. Further, the model holds that stress is largely functional in that it leads to *learning and improved coping ability.* It is this definition and theory of stress that most closely resembles that of anxiety.

Anxiety

According to Lyttle (1986), the term anxiety is derived from the Latin *anxietas*, meaning disquiet. Lyttle defines anxiety as 'the constellation of physical and psychological responses generated in response to threat, be the threat real or imagined'. He goes on to suggest that anxiety can result from a threat to an individual's self-esteem or from being placed in a position where the individual feels under pressure to perform beyond the level of their abilities; this is clearly in line with the transactional theory of stress. The phenomenon of anxiety is frequently subdivided into *trait* and *state* anxiety. Trait anxiety is described by Salmon (1993) as 'the disposition to become anxious in stressful situations'. *State* anxiety on the other hand is a *normal and positive response to perceived danger.* The associated fear mobilizes the sympathetic nervous system flight or fight response and again is perceived as functional as it increases alertness and, possibly, the individual's coping ability. It is therefore a useful state, having evolved to help us deal with potential threats. Salmon (1993) emphasizes the importance of ensuring that efforts by health care professionals to reduce anxiety should not eliminate 'processes that are psychologically beneficial'.

The differentiation between state and trait anxiety is important. The origins of *trait* anxiety are often extremely complex (Lyttle 1986) and individuals frequently *defend* against anxiety (thought to be concerned with preserving self-image and sometimes known as maladaptive coping) rather than *manage* the causes directly (adaptive coping). Miller (1987) describes these two coping styles in terms of people's need for information. He terms those who actively seek information as *monitors* – these are people who are trying to manage their anxiety. Individuals who prefer to try and extract themselves from the perceived stressful event, for example surgery, Miller terms as *blunters* – these are people who are defending against their anxiety. This theory has clear implications for information-giving in day surgery.

Additionally, it is quite common for individuals to fail to recognize that they are in fact anxious. If the source of their anxiety is not clear to the individual, the symptoms they are feeling can be interpreted as having an organic cause.

Learning Points

- *Trait anxiety* – the tendency to become anxious in stressful situations; individuals frequently *defend* against anxiety.
- *State anxiety* – a positive and normal response to threat; thought to be functional as it promotes coping ability and therefore the likelihood of *managing* anxiety.

Manifestations of Anxiety

Anxiety can manifest itself in both psychological and physiological symptoms, many of which may be familiar to you. Clearly the level of anxiety will influence the severity of the manifestations (Boxes 7.1 and 7.2).

It is perhaps not surprising that many individuals attribute these symptoms, especially those affecting the cardiovascular and respiratory systems, to a physical and possibly more sinister cause. Worrying about the possibility of serious physical disease will clearly increase the symptoms experienced.

Box 7.1 Pychological effects of anxiety (Bond 1986)

Inability to relax	Restlessness	Irritability
Poor concentration	Forgetfulness	Insomnia
Nightmares	Panic attacks	Depression
Feelings of insecurity	Feelings of tension	Fatigue

Box 7.2 Physiological effects of anxiety (Bond 1986)

- ***Cardiovascular system*** – tachycardia, palpitations, dropped beats, chest pain, flushing, faintness, blood pressure can be increased or decreased.
- ***Respiratory system*** – increased respirations, shortness of breath, yawning, sighing, tightness in chest.
- ***Gastro-intestinal system*** – nausea, vomiting, belching, diarrhoea, dyspepsia, 'butterflies', dry mouth, weight loss, anorexia or increased appetite, dysphagia, constipation.
- ***Urinary system*** – frequency, stress incontinence.
- ***Musculo-skeletal system*** – aches and pains, teeth clenching, increased muscular tension and weakness.
- ***Reproductive system*** – decreased libido, increased menstrual flow, increased dysmenorrhoea.
- ***Skin*** – perspiration, pallor, blushing, cold clammy palms.
- ***Nervous system*** – tension, headaches, blurred vision, tinnitus, tremor, clonic jerks, migraine.

The Sources of Pre-operative Anxiety

So what are the common causes of anxiety in surgical patients? Burden (1993) believes that all patients have the right to be anxious. As outlined at the start of the chapter, much state anxiety can be attributed to fear of the unknown. Swindale (1989) offers a useful framework for assessment of anxiety in patients having minor surgery. She identifies a number of influences on perception of anxiety (Fig. 7.2):

- from within the individual and their own sphere of experience
- from aspects perceived to be threatening about admission to hospital
- from factors inherent in the ward or unit environment.

Back in 1974, Franklin concluded that therapeutic discussion directed at relieving patient anxiety was virtually non-existent; as indicated in Chapter 4, perhaps we are still guilty of making too many 'reassuring noises'. Salmon (1993) argues that the provision of emotional support (i.e. giving patients the opportunity to put their fears into words and for these to be accepted, rather than countered with non-specific reassurance) will help to reduce patients feelings of helplessness in the face of threat. Assessment of anxiety therefore hinges on the ability to listen. There is evidence to suggest that patients with differing levels of pre-operative anxiety require different means of psychological preparation (Ridgeway & Matthews 1982, Hathaway 1986).

Assessing Anxiety

It seems important therefore to assess *levels* of anxiety, rather than simply its presence; only then can nursing interventions be individually tailored. In a seminal piece of work as early as 1958,

Figure 7.2 Possible variables affecting anxiety on admission (adapted from Swindale 1989)

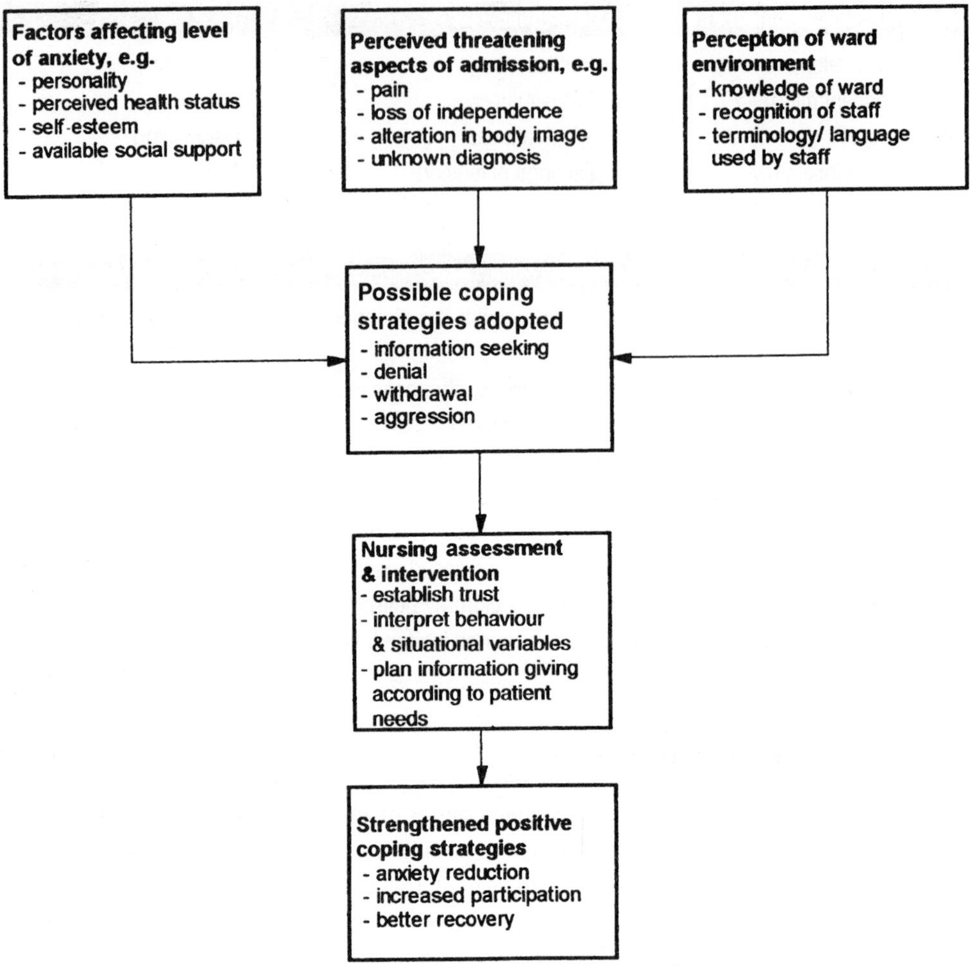

Janis was exploring the effects of pre-operative anxiety on postoperative recovery. His findings indicated that those individuals whose anxiety was either *extreme* or *absent* pre-operatively tended to experience a poor recovery. Janis concluded that 'realistic' (moderate) levels of anxiety facilitated positive coping ability and argued that patients in this position were able to plan for forthcoming events and sensations. However, as Salmon (1993) points out, at present there seems to be a more pervasive view amongst nurses that any anxiety is inherently harmful and should therefore be alleviated. This view appears to result in the delivery of a great deal of non-specific and often non-helpful 'reassurance'. Not only do nurses appear to overestimate the worries their

Learning Points

- Patients have a right to be anxious.
- Not all anxiety is harmful – ***moderate*** levels can help patients prepare for forthcoming events.
- ***Assessment*** is therefore vital to a tailored approach to anxiety management.

patients may have (Johnston 1982) they also tend to give the same 'anti-anxiety' care, regardless of its appropriateness to a particular individual.

The goal of pre-operative psychological care should *not* therefore be the elimination of anxiety; what Janis described as the *work of worry* and Salmon as *preparatory worry* is good for the individual; this equates with a moderate state of anxiety. It mobilizes resources, makes people more alert to dangers and aids readiness to learn. Nurses' responsibility should be geared towards assessment of the level of anxiety and then adopting one of a number of strategies; telling someone not to worry is not one of them. It should start with the nurse encouraging verbalization of fears and that requires skill (see Chapter 4 and care plan, Chapter 6). Salmon (1993) concludes that evidence related to anxiety and poor recovery is ambiguous. The use of measures such as circulating cortisol, catecholamines and ADH have not produced conclusive results. His research supports that of Janis, suggesting that only people with very low and very high anxiety levels have poorer recovery.

An individualized approach to anxiety assessment and reduction (when necessary) is vital when dealing with the different age groups encountered in day surgery. For instance, when children are scheduled for surgery, much is done to alleviate the child's distress, but what of the parents? Norris (1992) presents evidence that mothers of children having day surgery are more anxious, probably as a result of their greater responsibility in their child's care. She goes on to point out that presence of parents in the anaesthetic room should be common practice for all preschool children, which is likely to have beneficial effects on both child and parental anxiety. In addition, Ellerton and Merriam (1994 – a synopsis of the research is to be found in Chapter 5) argue that preparation of the *family* should be the goal of care.

Strategies for Preparing Patients Psychologically for Day Surgery

Much has been written and taught about the importance of psychological preparation of patients for anaesthetic and surgery. Regardless of how the preparation takes place, success hinges on the quality of the relationship between nurse and patient and honest communication: 'the greatest cure for fear is trust' (Kneedler & Dodge 1991). The most commonly utilized means of psychological preparation aimed at anxiety reduction fall into one of the following categories:

- non-specific (and often non-helpful) 'reassurance'
- planned procedural information
- sensory information
- attention control (distraction)
- cognitive coping strategies
- relaxation.

Non-specific Reassurance

It is interesting to examine the word 'reassurance'. A standard term in many care plans, the word is used to cover a number of non-specific nursing actions, directed towards *making patients feel better.* If patient anxiety is identified in a care plan, the outcome for nursing intervention is often simply *to reassure.* Often, there is no specific means of achieving this outcome identified in the care plan, beyond that of 'give explanations as necessary' or 'arrange for patient to see doctor'. But reassurance cannot be given, like you would give a hot drink. As discussed earlier in Chapter 4, these rather tired and meaningless statements about reassurance indicate a lack of individuality in care planning, but it need not necessarily be a true reflection of actual nursing intervention. However, if it is, and we suggest that this is probably the case, it may be a feature of uncertainty or discomfort on the part of nurses in dealing with patients' distress. That said, it may also reflect the continuing *over-emphasis* on routine physical aspects of patient preparation or preoccupation with organizational anomalies associated with a particular surgeon's operating list. Making sure the list 'runs smoothly' then assumes priority and becomes more important than meeting individual patient's needs. As a consequence, the lack of attention to psychological preparation can be *justified.*

It is interesting that many nurses argue that they would concern themselves more with psychological preparation, *if only they had the time.* But experience tells us that nurses in day surgery frequently *do* have 'time' – what is important for patient well-being and quality of care is how they choose to use that time.

Planned Procedural Information

Information on aspects of admission, the procedure and after care probably represents the most common form of preparation for surgery (Mitchell 1994). Most of the early research exploring the effects of information on anxiety reduction, pain perception and postoperative recovery, were evaluating this type of preparation, (e.g. Hayward 1975, Boore 1978). Hayward argued that essential information to be given pre-operatively should include:

- fasting times and rationale
- premedication and effects
- transfer to theatre
- induction
- recovery
- postoperative circumstances.

However, Summers (1984) found that up to 60% of this type of information was forgotten by patients, especially those who were very anxious. This view is supported by Burden (1993) who suggests that too many nurses believe that providing simple explanations is all that is required to relieve patients' anxiety; this is certainly not always the case. Another problem with procedural information is that the words that nurses use may have different meanings for the patients for whom the information is intended. Teasdale (1995) suggests that nurses should spend less time worrying about being accurate and precise and concentrate more on the context in which the information is given. Similarly, information leaflets for patients may use accurate words and sentences but when they are read at home with the family, the context has changed and so therefore can the meaning be changed.

Giving procedural information is also of little value if no other strategy is adopted to assess and deal with raised anxiety levels; this reinforces our earlier recommendation for assessment of *levels* of pre-operative anxiety.

Ridgeway and Mathews (1982) study of pre-operative anxiety adopted a different approach. One group of patients were taught cognitive coping methods (e.g. concentrating on the benefits of proposed surgery) whilst the other group received comprehensive procedural information. The results indicated that although the latter group knew more about their surgery, the former group had the better recovery. According to Hathaway (1986) procedural information can be useful when patients' anxiety levels are low to moderate, but when they are high, sensory and psychological information are the more effective options.

Children over 2 years old require a simple explanation of the anaesthetic procedure with close attention to the words used. Separate children's pre-admission assessment sessions are a useful means of providing information for parents and children (see Chapter 5) and are often run on a Saturday morning. Pellet (1990) describes a possible programme for such a 'Saturday club', indicating that both parents and children benefit from the relaxed, yet informative style.

Sensory Information

The provision of sensory information helps patients rehearse for the experience of surgery (Dodds 1993). It is based on the supposition that if sensory input (i.e. what patients may see, hear, feel, taste or smell during the experience) does not fit with a mental image of some previous experience (known as a schema), anxiety levels will rise. Some examples of sensory information would be the changes in temperature within the department, the feeling of cold or tingling in their arm during an intravenous injection, the smells in the anaesthetic room, etc. – sensations that may cause alarm if not prepared for (Mitchell 1994). The combination of appropriate sensory information with other types of psychological preparation, such as promoting cognitive coping strategies, can be most effective (Johnston *et al.* 1978, Ridgeway & Mathews 1982).

Attention Control (Distraction)

This strategy is only really of benefit if the individual wishes to be distracted or if they are too young to realize that is the intention. Clearly, distracting children by encouraging play or watching television or video is an example of such a strategy, but will only really be effective when the child is quite young. In ideal circumstances, all children's day surgery would take place on a paediatric day unit (Brykczynska 1995), but it is more common to have a designated area on a general day unit (see Chapter 12). A special children's room, appropriately decorated and kitted out with *safe* and suitable toys, books, comics and games is essential; close liaison with nursing staff on the hospital's paediatric wards and play therapist if they have one, is a must. *Play preparation* for surgery helps to familiarize children with who is who and the words used to describe their forthcoming surgery (Chandler 1994). As the number of dedicated children's lists increase with planned admission times, the time spent waiting for the procedure should decrease. Children should be encouraged to have their blanket or 'teddy' or other meaningful toy or comforter with them, who can also undergo some of the same preparation, for example an identity band.

For adults, providing means of distraction, such as a range of up-to-date magazines and journals is important, as patients, once prepared, frequently have to wait for considerable periods of time before their surgery. It is precisely during this time that anxiety can be at its highest and often when there is time for nurses to do more than to *instruct* patients to sit back, relax and read a magazine!

Cognitive Coping Strategies

In some ways, this strategy for anxiety reduction is akin to distraction, but one in which patients themselves retain control. Cognitive coping strategies are based on the transactional theory of stress (see earlier in the chapter) and the premise that the human brain is able to mediate between the stressor and the response. This theory of stress holds that stress is a result of a mismatch between the demands the individual believes have been placed upon them and their perceived ability to cope. When admitted to hospital the person, to some extent, loses their individuality and is forced to take on a new, and often more passive role.

Cognitive coping strategies are simple exercises that can be taught to patients in order that they can regain some control over this new situation. For example, patients may be encouraged to *think* of a more 'normal' situation in which they felt they coped well. They are then encouraged to identify what it was about that situation that allowed them to cope more effectively and the skills they used to achieve the result. It is then suggested to patients that they concentrate on these skills and behaviours, rather than on how they are dealing with this present stressful event. Although the effectiveness of such strategies is difficult to assess (Mitchell 1994), the fact that nurses are spending time with patients, in teaching these exercises, is likely to be positively welcomed. In common with all strategies, assessment of levels of anxiety is essential.

Relaxation

A number of studies over the past 20 years have indicated that relaxation can reduce anxiety and enhance postoperative recovery (e.g. Levin *et al.* 1987, Edelmann 1992). Most of us can think of a time when we have either tried deep breathing exercises ourselves or suggested that patients try them. Regardless of the difficulty in assessing the outcome of such a strategy, the simple answer may be that, in common with cognitive coping strategies, relaxation helps us and our patients feel more *in control.* We are aware that the response to the suggestion that structured relaxation may be of benefit to some patients pre-operatively will be that you do not have the time! But there are a number of ways that relaxation can be taught to a *group* of patients, if they are interested, *at booked pre-admission assessment.* The patients are encouraged to practise simple techniques at home and especially on the day prior to admission, when it is estimated that state anxiety is at its highest (Johnston 1980). One study that sought to explore the impact of relaxation on patients scheduled for day surgery is outlined below in Box 7.3.

There is little doubt that anxiety assessment and management is an important aspect of the nurses role in day surgery. Much of the success of strategies such as those described hinges on nurses' willingness to engage in meaningful interactions with patients and to make the best possible use of available time prior to surgery. This applies also to theatre-based nurses on an integrated day surgery unit; although they are in an ideal position to visit patients pre-operatively, very few choose to do so (see Chapter 9).

Finally, there is one more point to make in relation to the subject of anxiety. How can we possibly fulfil the requirements of *informed consent* if we do not address patient anxiety?

Box 7.3 Research study

In a study carried out on a day surgery unit in North Wales, Markland and Hardy (1993) were keen to examine the impact of a brief relaxation procedure on pre-operative state anxiety, and induction and maintenance of anaesthesia. A convenience sample of 21 patients took part in the study (17 males and 4 females) who were to undergo a variety of procedures, e.g. vasectomy, cystoscopy, excision of breast lump, varicose vein surgery. All patients consented freely to take part, received routine pre-operative care and standard procedural information and were randomly allocated to one of three groups:

Group 1 – patients listened to a tape-recorded relaxation session on a personal stereo. The tape lasted approximately 20 min and included a number of different techniques, such as attention to body parts and breathing and increasing and releasing tension in muscle groups.

Group 2 – patients listened to a 20 min tape-recorded short story. The story was described as 'fairly innocuous and unlikely to arouse excitement'. As such, this treatment constituted attention control.

Group 3 – patients were simply asked to lie on their beds and wait (what most patients on most day units experience) – this was the 'no treatment' control group.

The same researcher measured state anxiety of all 21 patients using Spielbergers State–Trait anxiety inventory and recorded heart rate and blood pressure before and after 'treatment'. These interventions were timed to take place within the 40 min prior to surgery.

On arrival in the anaesthetic room the same anaesthetist treated all the patients with a standard regime and recorded:

- amount of sodium thiopentone required to induce loss of eyelid reflex
- time taken in seconds to achieve loss of chin and swallowing reflexes
- the measure of maintenance (mean concentration per minute of isoflurane) from placing patient on table to end of procedure
- linear analogue measures of 'difficulty' of both induction and maintenance of anaesthesia.

- Only Group 1 had a significant reduction in state anxiety on all measures of anxiety (at post-test).
- Group 3 (control) state anxiety scores were higher at post-test which reinforces the theory that **anxiety increases with waiting unless specific intervention occurs**.
- Both experimental groups (1 & 2) demonstrated benefits for anaesthetic requirements when compared with the control (Group 3).
- Group 1 had the advantage over Group 2 in terms of reported ease/difficulty of maintenance.

Although by no means perfect in terms of design, the study offers evidence of the effectiveness of relaxation on state anxiety.

Informed Consent

It is perhaps worth exploring the issue of consent here, especially as in day surgery some considerable time can elapse between obtaining consent and the surgery actually taking place. According to Hewetson (1994), health professionals' knowledge and understanding of consent is, at best, incomplete. She argues that this situation suggests not only that lip service is being paid to central concepts of autonomy and partnership, but that nurses and clinicians may be exposing themselves to civil and criminal actions.

From a moral position, informed consent has two fundamental components – *information giving* and *consent to treatment*; the first requiring communication skills and the latter, understanding (McLean & Maher 1993).

Hewetson outlines the three basic criteria for consent:

- *capacity* – this the capability of the individual to understand the proposed treatment,
- *disclosure of information:*
  (1) the individual must understand the nature of the proposed treatment in broad terms, and why it has been prescribed
  (2) disclosure or non-disclosure of potential side-effects – the individual must understand the principal benefits and risks and the consequences of *not* having the treatment
- *voluntariness* – consent is to be voluntary; this cannot be guaranteed if the individual is under the influence of sedation.

It is worth remembering that consent can be given verbally, in writing or by implication and all are legally valid (Dimond 1995), but *only when these three components are present.*

A useful view of consent that recognizes that it is far more than getting a patient to sign a form and emphasizes the relationship between nurse or doctor and patient is put forward by Downie and Calman (1987). They see consent:

- as a legal device designed to protect individuals and their autonomy
- as legal protection for professionals
- as an extension of a relationship that is based on trust.

Informed consent therefore relates not just to participation in research or consent to treatment, *but to any relationship between the health care professional and a patient.* This understanding of consent raises certain responsibilities for nurses and doctors and the process must therefore:

- respect individual autonomy
- protect the patient
- avoid untruths, duress or anxiety
- promote rational decision-making.

Informed consent for a procedure is specific to that procedure and that individual patient (Burden 1993).The written consent form, as Wicker (1991) reminds us, is simply an indication that at the time of signing, the individual gave their consent; it is not a guarantee that the individual still feels that way. In the same way, when patients present themselves on the day surgery unit, it is not safe to assume they are in effect implying consent. Ideally, the surgeon should check and once more explain the nature of the surgery with its benefits and limitations when they visit patients prior to surgery. The information provided must be sufficient to allow an informed decision to be made, though some clinicians may think that they know what is best for their patients and may believe that giving too much information may not be in their best interests. But it is essentially wrong to make that assumption . Although there is no requirement in English law that all possible side-effects must be made clear, as Henry and Pashley (1990) point out, 'laws do not in themselves provide moral justification'.

We have included some recommended reading at the end of this chapter for all staff who are unsure of their knowledge regarding this important issue.

Learning Points

- Many health professionals knowledge and understanding of consent is incomplete or inaccurate.
- Informed consent requires both information-giving and consent to treatment.
- Unresolved anxiety will interfere with learning and understanding.
- The ability to give consent hinges on three basic criteria:
  (1) capacity
  (2) disclosure of information
  (3) voluntariness.
- Patients have the fundamental right to refuse treatment or surgery.

Aspects of Physical Preparation

It is clear that patients undergoing day surgery require physical preparation with the same focus on safety as those on inpatient wards. Day surgery patients will be receiving some form of anaesthesia (see Chapter 8) and the preparation and care they require should be based upon the known and possible effects of the selected anaesthetic, *not* the established routines that characterize automatic and non-critical practice. There is little doubt that pre-operative care represents an area of practice that is still in need of more rational thought and flexibility. The advent and growth of day surgery, improved anaesthetic techniques and the developing role of nurses in the specialty should be providing sufficient stimulus to continue to challenge the more ritualized aspects of practice and provide safe, individualized and research-based care. We now look briefly at two aspects of pre-operative care, fasting and skin preparation, and present some guidelines for good practice.

Fasting

Anaesthetists in day surgery have been at the forefront of research into patient fasting times over the last decade, and current practice represents a major step forward from the times of ritual starvation of patients, often for up to 12 h. In 1972, Hamilton-Smith's large-scale study into fasting times for patients involved nurses and anaesthetists and found considerable variation in fasting times ranging from 4 to 12 h. The majority of nurses in the study failed to understand the essential reasons of fasting, demonstrated little evidence of flexibility and planning and apparently preferred to err on the side of safety. A small-scale replication of this work completed by Thomas (1987) suggested that the same practices were alive and well 15 years later. Hung's study in 1992 found likewise and suggested that fasting times were still being planned to suit nurses' convenience rather than the interests of patients.

Excessive fasting has potentially deleterious effects on patients well-being. Goodwin *et al.* (1991), in a study of day surgery patients suggest that pre-operative hunger and thirst may contribute to postoperative nausea and vomiting, while Neill (1995) presents evidence that prolonged fasting in children increases parental and child anxiety and distress on waking from anaesthetic. In addition, there is an increased likelihood of hypoglycaemia, dehydration and nausea. Neill suggests that there are a number of reasons why parents fast their children for longer than necessary, making clear instructions and rationale for safe fasting times essential for parental co-operation. Thornes (1991) cites evidence that indicates that parents frequently starve themselves 'in sympathy' with their children, which may lead to 'physiological consequences that can exacerbate their anxiety'.

In fact, all patients must be given clear and unambiguous instructions regarding the need for and what constitutes fasting. In a study of 116 patients' knowledge of anaesthesia and peri-operative care, nearly 30% thought fasting referred only to food (Hume *et al.* 1994).

During fasting, gastric secretions of up to 50 ml per hour continue to be produced (Goodwin *et al.* 1991). Anxiety not only increases gastric secretion, but reduces the rate at which the stomach empties. In addition, the rate of gastric emptying varies between individuals and according to the *type* of fluid and food ingested. These factors must be taken into consideration when assessing the necessary fasting time. Studies suggest that healthy patients who consume clear fluids 2 – 4 h pre-operatively have no greater residual gastric volume than those who have fasted for much longer (Miller *et al.* 1983, Maltby *et al.* 1986). Consequently, a more rational period of fasting for both adults and children is now being adopted (Strunin 1993, Phillips *et al.* 1994). As a guide to good practice, patients should be asked to:

- not eat solids within 4 h of surgery
- drink normally until within 4 h of surgery
- drink up to $\frac{1}{2}$ pint (275 ml) of fluid – juice, tea or coffee up to within 2 h of surgery. We advise that for children under the age of 10 years, the quantity be reduced to a 100 ml (a cup).

Skin Preparation

Early assumptions that removing hair (and thereby potentially harmful micro-organisms) from the site of operation would reduce the incidence of infection have long been questioned. Close skin shaving causes micro skin abrasions and a fertile area for bacterial growth, thereby *increasing* the risk of infection (Alexander *et al.* 1983). It is not the removal of the hair that is the problem, but the disruption of the epidermis. However, it is clearly necessary for the surgeon to see the operation site, and therefore, removal of some body hair is necessary. Depilatory creams have been used with some success (Lancet 1983), although they are costly, skin reactions are quite common and the practice appears to carry the same wound-infection risk as shaving (Winfield 1986). Electric clippers have also been used; these leave the epidermis intact, but are expensive to purchase, maintain and sterilize.

In day surgery units, the responsibility for pre-operative skin cleansing and preparation lies with the patients. Although written information usually requests them to bathe prior to admission, the optimum timing of that bath or shower is often not made explicit and specific instructions about washing are rarely given. In addition, when shaving is required, verbal or written instructions largely fail to stipulate *when* it is best to shave, or give enough consideration to the patient's mobility, dexterity or available equipment. The razor in the bathroom cabinet may be '*the best a man can get*', but it may not be the best for a pubic shave! Similarly, the thought of shaving the pubic area must strike terror into many people, young or old. Patients should be reassured that if they, or a relative is unable to manage the shave, assistance on the day of operation will be available. Clearly, the most important issue here is a policy for skin preparation that is based on a rational approach and available research.

As a guide to good practice, verbal and written instructions for patients regarding skin preparation must be clear and unambiguous. Such information should include timing of a bath or shower (as near to admission as possible), when to shave if required (the morning of admission at the time of bath or shower), and the extent of the required shave. Patients should be provided with skin prep razors at the time of pre-admission assessment if necessary and advised to wet shave as this decreases the likelihood of cuts and abrasions. They should also be advised not to apply any cream or lotions to the area once it has been shaved.

The Pre-operative Check List

The completion of a pre-operative check list is a nursing requirement, not a patient problem. Completion of this check list will not in itself achieve a reduction in patient anxiety, nor will it reduce the likelihood of postoperative complications, as both of these are frequently claimed to do in patients' care plans. There are, however, specific elements of pre-operative management that help to minimize risks and it is clearly good practice to have a recognized and simple means of checking that all of these necessary preparations have been completed prior to patient's transfer to theatre. That said, it is equally important that items on the checklist are reviewed periodically to ensure that their rationale remains appropriate. For instance, it has always been common practice to remove patients' dentures prior to general anaesthesia. The practice assumes that all dentures tend to be loose fitting and easily displaced and fails to take into account the effects of removal on self-image or the common use of denture fixative. Current research is looking at the implications of leaving good fitting dentures in place during anaesthesia. A check list (Fig. 7.3) commonly covers aspects of pre-operative preparation.

It is essential that completion of a safety checklist such as this does not become yet another example of ritualized practice; it is completed for a purpose and the vital concept of patient safety must remain paramount during any pre-operative preparation. The anaesthetist must be informed immediately of any concerns about patient fitness (see Chapter 8). Sharing responsibility for pre-operative care may result in vital aspects of care not being addressed or information not being recorded. One trained nurse must take responsibility for ensuring that:

- Information gathered at pre-admission assessment is available and any changes in circumstances or fitness are recorded and reported to the anaesthetist. This should include current weight, blood pressure, any current medication, known allergies, relevant medical history, smoking habits and dentition.
- Patients undergo rational and safe preparation on the day of surgery and all relevant documentation is completed and signed.
- All information is documented in the care plan (for example, see Fig. 7.4).

Clearly, the most effective means of achieving this and the requirements of the concept of the named nurse, is to adopt a system of primary nursing, whereby all registered nurses assume explicit and signed accountability for a group of patients from admission to discharge and beyond to telephone follow-up. However, regardless of differences in organization of nursing care, what is important here is the notion of *signed accountability.* All relevant

Figure 7.3 The pre-operative checklist

Element **– normally, these should be removed**	***Rationale***
Does the patient have any:	
■ contact lenses?	*Can get lost, or potentially cause corneal damage*
■ dentures?	*If loose fitting, could dislodge and occlude airway*
■ hair grips?	*Can damage scalp through pressure*
■ jewellery?	*Items, especially rings with stones can cause skin damage through pressure, or become damaged. Taping of jewellery* ***does not*** *protect the patient from electrical injury! A wedding ring need only be taped if the patient wishes to keep it on, but it is loose and at risk of falling off*
■ make up?	*Can mask changes in skin colour*
■ prostheses?	*Can be dislodged/ misplaced*

Element **– these should be checked and noted**	***Rationale***
Does the patient wear a hearing aid?	*If yes, the device should always remain with the patient to aid communication*
Does the patient have any allergies?	*Principally refers to metals, drugs and dressing tapes – may come in contact with allergen during procedure. People with allergy to eggs, should not receive* ***propofol***
Are medical notes and X-rays available?	*Ensures match between patient identity and procedure. Provides information regarding past medical history*
Are relevant pathology reports available?	*Provides confirmation of test results/ diagnosis*
Is the consent form signed?	*Should provide confirmation of informed consent*
Is the operation site shaved (if necessary)?	*To allow good visual field*
Operation site marked (if necessary)?	*To ensure correct procedure*
Is the identification band correct?	*To ensure match between patient identity and procedure*
Does the patient have any dental crowns or bridgework?	*Provides information for anaesthetist so as to prevent damage to dental work*
Has the patient emptied their bladder?	*To prevent voiding of urine during anaesthetic and bladder damage in pelvic surgery*
Has any premedication been given?	*Confirms drug, dose and time of administration*
For children	***Rationale***
Has local anaesthetic cream been applied? Note time and number of sites?	*Significantly reduces pain of intravenous induction; should be applied 1 h pre-operatively*
Has parent been supplied with overshoes and gown?	*Prevents delay and potential distress on transfer to theatre*

Figure 7.4 Pre-operative care plan (specimen)

Potential patient problem	Goal/outcome	Nursing actions
Lack of knowledge of own role in preoperative preparation	**Patient is able to describe their role accurately and carry out specific preparation with confidence**	• Provide a suitable environment for assessment, taking into account factors in the patient or carer that may influence concentration and/or learning • Assess patients' (and relatives' if appropriate) present knowledge and understanding of condition requiring treatment and the nature of surgical intervention • Assist understanding with explanation of procedure in straightforward terms as necessary • Provide information on preoperative preparation required, to include fasting and skin preparation when necessary, and supplement with relevant written material • Assess understanding through questioning and discussion, and answer any further questions • On day of surgery, ensure patient has completed necessary preparation
Anxiety related to admission and forthcoming surgery	**Patient is able to express their concerns and feels more calm and comfortable**	• Encourage patient to assess level of their anxiety using analogue scale if appropriate, and to identify their usual coping strategies • Encourage patient to express the source of their concerns • Provide further procedural information if patient feels their anxiety is controlled • If anxiety is increased, provide sensory information, e.g. sights, smells, feelings associated with procedure to help patient 'rehearse' for event • Provide distraction through reading material if appropriate

You will see that both the nursing actions in relation to the above problems could be further divided into pre-admission assessment and day of surgery assessment if appropriate. You may think that more problems should be documented; that is an individual decision. A second sheet following the same outline would be necessary for documenting other problems identified at assessment. You will also see that we have not identified specific elements of pre-operative preparation (i.e. safety precautions) under patient problems. The reason is simple; they are not patient problems. They are nursing responsibilities, and are best kept on a separate check list.

Potential patient problem	Goal/outcome	Nursing actions

information can then be passed from nurse to anaesthetist or operating department practitioner without a third party being involved. As Norris (1992) points out, the more people involved in a patient's care, the more chance there is of conflicting information being given, or vital information being omitted.

Summary

We must provide quality pre-operative care that is based on individualized assessment of psychological needs and a clear understanding of the principles of safety in relation to the administration of anaesthesia. In order to achieve these goals, the following factors require close consideration:

- the number of patients on any one operating list
- provision of staggered admission times
- quality prebooked pre-admission assessment for all patients
- rational pre-operative preparation protocols and written patient information
- simple nursing documentation and, most of all,
- skilled and motivated staff.

The preparation of patients for surgery involves elements of both psychological and physical care. The often quite rapid throughout in modern day surgery units can in itself be a source of anxiety for patients as they can perceive themselves to be merely objects on a conveyor belt. Similarly, the speed with which patients often need to be admitted and prepared can militate against the provision of more individualized care. Although we recognize that time can sometimes be at a premium, there are many opportunities for nurses to provide more individualized and effective psychological support for patients.

Key Points

- Stressors such as fear of surgery or possible diagnosis induce neuro-endocrine responses that may have undesirable consequences for anaesthetic induction and maintenance and patients' recovery.
- Day surgery patients are considered to be amongst the most anxious of all surgical patients.
- Not all anxiety is harmful; moderate levels can motivate patients to learn about their condition and surgery and prepare for the experience.
- Anxiety is at its highest on the day before admission and during the time between admission and induction of anaesthesia; the latter is a time when more effective support could be provided.
- Assessment of level of anxiety, not merely its presence, is essential.

- There are a number of different strategies for the reduction of anxiety; the choice hinges on accurate assessment; the use of non-verbal skills, the provision of sensory information and teaching structured relaxation are amongst the most effective, yet are undervalued and under-used.
- Physical preparation of patients for day surgery should be based on principles of safety and rational protocols.
- Quality patient information, both verbal and written is fundamental to safe preparation.
- Ensuring safe preparation and effective patient support is best facilitated by primary nursing.

Recommended Reading

Davies, N. (1994) **Legal Aspects of Day Case Surgery.** In Whitwam, J. G. (Ed) (1994) *Day Case Anaesthesia & Sedation.* Oxford: Blackwell Scientific Publications

A useful short chapter covering a number of legal issues in day surgery

Dimond, B. (1995) **Legal Aspects of Nursing** (Second Edition). London: Prentice-Hall

This is an excellent text to dip into for specific information; we particularly recommend chapter 7 on consent and informing the patient

Hewetson, G. (1994) **Ignorance is not bliss – informed consent.** *British Journal of Theatre Nursing* **4**(9): 14–16

A useful overview of moral and legal dimensions of consent

References

Alexander, J. W., Fischer, J. E., Boyajian, M., Palaiquist, J. and Morris, M. J. (1983) **The influence of hair removal methods on wound infections.** *Archives of Surgery* **118**: 347–351.

Bond, M. (1986) **Stress & Self-Awareness – A guide for nurses.** London: Heinemann.

Boore, J. (1978) **Prescription for recovery: the effects of preoperative preparation of surgical patients on post-operative stress, recovery and infection.** London: RCN.

Brykczynska, G. (1995) **Ethics of day surgery for children.** *Surgical Nurse* **8**(1): 11–13.

Burden, N. (1993) **Ambulatory Surgery Nursing.** Philadelphia: Saunders.

Chandler, K. (1994) **Play Preparation for Surgery.** *Surgical Nurse* **7**(4): 14–16.

Dimond, B. (1995) **Legal Aspects of Nursing** (Second Edition). London: Prentice-Hall.

Dodds, F. (1993) **Access to the coping strategies: managing anxiety in elective surgical patients.** *Professional Nurse* **9**(1): 45–52.

Downie, R. S. and Calman, K. C. (1987) **Healthy Respect: Ethics in Health Care.** London: Faber & Faber.

Edelmann, R. J. (1992) **Anxiety Theory, Research & Intervention in Clinical & Health Psychology.** Chichester: Wiley.

Ellerton, M. L. and Merriam, C. (1994) **Preparing children and families psychologically for day surgery: an evaluation.** *Journal of Advanced Nursing* **19**: 1057–1062.

Franklin, B. L. (1974) **Patient anxiety on admission to hospital.** London: RCN.

Goodwin, A. P. L., Rowe, W. L., Ogg, T. W. and Samaan, A. (1991) **Oral fluids prior to day surgery.** *Anaesthesia* **46**: 1066–1068.

Hamilton-Smith, S. (1972) **Nil by mouth?** London: RCN.

Hathaway, D. (1986) **Effect of preoperative instruction on postoperative outcomes: a meta-analysis.** *Nursing Research* **35**(5): 269–275.

Hayward, J. (1975) **Information – a prescription against pain.** London: RCN.

Henry, I. C. and Pashley, G. (1990) **Health Ethics.** Lancaster: Quay.

Hewetson, G. (1994) **Ignorance is not bliss – informed consent.** *British Journal of Theatre Nursing* **4**(9): 14–16.

Hume, M. A., Kennedy, B. and Ashbury, A. J. (1994) **Patient knowledge of anaesthesia and perioperative care.** *Anaesthesia* **49**: 715–718.

Hung, P. (1992) **Preoperative fasting.** *Nursing Times* **82**(10): 64–68.

Janis, I. L. (1958) **Psychological Stress.** New York: Wiley.

Johnston, J. E., Rice, V. H., Fuller, S. S. and Endress, M. P. (1978) **Sensory information, instruction on coping strategy and recovery from surgery.** *Research in Nursing & Health* **1**: 4–17.

Johnston, M. (1980) **Anxiety in surgical patients.** *Psychological Medicine* **10**: 145–152.

Johnston, M. (1982) **Recognition of patients worries by nurses and other patients.** *British Journal of Clinical Psychology* **21**: 255–261.

Kneedler, J. A. and Dodge, G. H. (1991) **Peri-operative Patient Care – The nursing perspective** (Second Edition). Boston: Jones & Bartlett.

Lancet (Ed) (1983) **Preoperative depilation.** *Lancet* **83**(1): 1311.

Lazarus, R. S. (1976) **Psychological Stress and the Coping Process.** New York: McGraw-Hill.

Levin, R. F., Malloy, G. B. and Hyman, R. B. (1987) **Nursing management of postoperative pain: use of relaxation techniques with female cholecystectomy patients.** *Journal of Advanced Nursing* **12**: 463–472.

Lyttle, J. (1986) **Mental Disorder: Its care and treatment.** London: Baillière Tindall.

Maltby, A. R., Sutherland, A. D., Sale, J. P. and Schaffer, E. A. (1986) **Pre-operative oral fluids: Is a five hour fast justified prior to elective surgery?** *Anaesthesia & Analgesia* **65**: 1112–1116.

Markland, D. and Hardy, L. (1993) Anxiety, relaxation and anaesthesia for day-case surgery. *British Journal of Clinical Psychology* **32**: 493–504.

McLean, S. and Maher, G. (1993) **Medicine, Morals and the Law.** London: Gower.

Miller, M., Wishart, H. Y. and Nimmo, W. S. (1983) **Gastric contents at induction of anaesthesia. Is a 4 hour fast necessary?** *British Journal of Anaesthesia* **55**: 1185–1188.

Miller, S. M. (1987) **Monitoring and blunting: validation of a questionnaire to assess style of information-seeking under threat.** *Journal of Personal & Social Psychology* **52**(2): 345–353.

Mitchell, M. (1994) **Day surgery: preoperative and postoperative psychological nursing care.** *Surgical Nurse* **7**(3): 22–25.

Neill, S. (1995) **Fasting for day surgery: the parental role.** *Paediatric Nursing* **7**(2): 20–23.

Norris, E. (1992) **Care of the paediatric day-surgery patient.** *British Journal of Nursing* **1**(11): 547–551.

Pellet, J. (1990) **General anaesthesia.** *Surgical Nurse* **3**(5): 21–26.

Phillips, S., Daborn, A. K. and Hatch, D. J. (1994) **Preoperative fasting for paediatric anaesthesia.** *British Journal of Anaesthesia* **73**: 529–536.

Ridgeway, V. and Mathews, A. (1982) **Psychological preparation of patients for surgery: a comparison of methods.** *British Journal of Clinical Psychology* **21**: 271–280.

Salmon, P. (1993) **The reduction of anxiety in surgical patients: an important nursing task or the medicalisation of preparatory worry?** *International Journal of Nursing Studies* **30**(4): 323–330.

Selye, H. (1976) **The Stress of Life.** New York: McGraw-Hill.

Strunin, L. (1993) **How long should patients fast before surgery? Time for new guidelines.** *British Journal of Anaesthesia* **70**: 1–3.

Summers, R. (1984) **Should patients be told more?** *Nursing Mirror* **159**(7): 16–20.

Swindale, J. E. (1989) **The nurses role in giving preoperative information to reduce anxiety in patients admitted to hospital for minor surgery.** *Journal of Advanced Nursing* **14**: 899–905.

Teasdale, K. (1995) **The nurse's role in anxiety management.** *Professional Nurse* **10**(8): 509–512.

Thomas, E. A. (1987) **Preoperative fasting; a question of routine?** *Nursing Times* **83**(49): 46–47.

Thornes, R. (1991) **All in a day's work.** *Paediatric Nursing* February: 7–8.

Wicker, C. P. (1991) **Legal responsibilities of the nurse 3. Assault and consent.** *Surgical Nurse* **4**(1): 16–17.

Wilson-Barnett, J. (1980) **Prevention and alleviation of stress in patients.** *Nursing* **10**: 432–436.

Winfield, U. (1986) **Too close a shave?** *Nursing Times* **82**(10): 64–68.

Chapter 8 Anaesthesia and pain control

Overview

This chapter provides an introduction to the various types of anaesthesia used in day surgery, including local anaesthesia, general anaesthesia and sedation techniques. The requirements for safe preparation of patients for anaesthesia are reviewed and the anaesthetist's perspective on pre-admission assessment presented. The management of the patient in theatre and recovery and the monitoring required are discussed. The management of pain intra-operatively and postoperatively is reviewed and the choice of analgesic drugs, techniques of administration and new developments in this field is covered in depth. Techniques for the assessment of pain experienced by patients are presented and the place of audit considered.

Chapter Focus

- The concept of anaesthesia
- Defining sedation and anaesthesia
- Requirements for assessing patients for anaesthesia
- Techniques of anaesthesia
- Monitoring requirements
- Recovery techniques and assessment
- Assessment and management of pain

Introduction

It is interesting to note that the first successful demonstration of general anaesthesia was by William Morton (using ether) at Massachusetts General Hospital in October 1846 whilst the first successful use of local anaesthesia was not for another 20 years by Dr Carl Koller (using topical cocaine) in Vienna.

Three basic types of anaesthesia will be seen in day surgery

- sedation techniques
- local anaesthesia
- general anaesthesia.

Sedation is included in this chapter as it is a technique often seen in day surgery units that include endoscopy facilities and chair dental sessions. It is, however, important to differentiate between what is sedation as opposed to general anaesthesia. The Wylie Report (1981) defines sedation as

> A technique in which the use of a drug or drugs produces a state of depression of the central nervous system enabling treatment to be carried out, but during which verbal contact with the patient is maintained.

The critical wording here is *during which verbal contact with the patient is maintained*, any situation where contact with the patient is lost then comes under the definition of general anaesthesia given below.

Anaesthesia literally means *loss of sensation* therefore general anaesthesia can be defined as *any technique in which a drug or combination of drugs produces loss of sensation and loss of consciousness, as defined by failure to respond to verbal command*. There is no place for terms or techniques such as heavy sedation, as these carry a significant risk of producing general anaesthesia. Patients who lose consciousness may develop airway obstruction and be at risk of ventilatory and/or circulatory arrest (The Royal College of Anaesthetists & The Royal College of Radiologists 1992)

Learning Points

- ***Sedation*** – a technique in which the use of a drug or drugs produces a state of depression of the central nervous system enabling treatment to be carried out, but during which verbal contact with the patient is maintained
- ***General anaesthesia*** – any technique in which a drug or combination of drugs produces loss of sensation and loss of consciousness, as defined by failure to respond to verbal command

Sedation Techniques

For many years sedation and sedo-analgesia techniques have been utilized in dental practice and endoscopy services. Concern about deaths occurring in dental surgeries (Coplans & Curson 1982) led to several reports (Wylie Report 1981, Poswillo Report 1990) which made strong recommendations about monitoring and the use of both these techniques and general anaesthesia in this area. Standards of sedation and monitoring for gastro-intestinal endoscopy were published in 1991 (Bell *et al.* 1991). This latter article should be read by all staff involved in endoscopy procedures as it provides an extensive list of recommendations that include:

- safety and monitoring
- resuscitation equipment and drugs
- resuscitation training
- airway management equipment
- nurse to monitor patient throughout
- minimum dosage of drugs
- availability of specific antagonists
- the use of cannula in 'at risk' patients
- the use of oxygen
- continuation of monitoring in recovery.

Despite these developments doubts have been raised about the safety of sedation techniques in endoscopy and indeed it is suggested that the mortality compares unfavourably to that expected

Box 8.1 Pharmacology of diazepam and midazolam

Diazepam

This drug is not water soluble and is available in two preparations. Standard diazepam is dissolved in a mixture of propylene glycol, ethyl alcohol and sodium benzoate in benzoic acid which contributes to a high incidence of patients experiencing pain on injection and phlebitis following its use. The advent of Diazemuls which is a commercial preparation of diazepam in an oil-in-water emulsion similar to Intralipid has reduced the incidence of these problems. The intravenous dosage for sedation is around 0.2 mg kg^{-1} (reduced in shocked and elderly patients). It has an extremely long half-life (20–50 h) and unfortunately is metabolized into components that are also active sedatives.

Midazolam

This is a water-soluble drug that causes far fewer problems on intravenous injection. It has a half-life of around 2 h and it has largely taken over from diazepam because of these features. Dosage for sedation is around 0.07 mg kg^{-1} (indications for reduction as above). It is believed that there is an incidence of people who are slow to metabolize this drug.

from general anaesthesia (Charlton 1995). Increased use of monitoring has been shown to improve outcome in patients undergoing anaesthesia. It is therefore important for all staff to remember that the use of monitoring (a trained nurse must be present and the use of a pulse oximeter is a minimum requirement) and supplemental oxygen should also improve outcome in patients undergoing endoscopy. Sedation should be achieved by the use of a single agent (see sedo-analgesia later), the most popular agents in endoscopy being the benzodiazepines – diazepam and midazolam. These drugs have quite different pharmacological profiles.

Sedo-analgesia

This refers to the practice of combining an analgesic drug such as pethidine or morphine with one of the benzodiazepines. This practice is now discouraged in dental practice (Poswillo 1990) due to the risks of inducing general anaesthesia and respiratory depression though it may well still be used in some endoscopy services.

The requirements for recovery following sedation techniques should not be forgotten. Patients should be nursed and monitored in a suitably equipped recovery area and managed as for recovery from general anaesthesia (see later in chapter). Similar criteria for discharge from the recovery area should also be used.

Learning Points

- Sedation techniques have considerable inherent dangers.
- Patients undergoing sedation should be monitored and given supplemental oxygen.
- Sedo-analgesic techniques increase the risk of respiratory depression.

Local Anaesthesia

We have already learned that local anaesthesia was used some 20 years after the first successful general anaesthetics. Dr Koller in Vienna first used cocaine as a topical local anaesthetic for eye surgery, but it is interesting to note, however, that the idea for this came from his famous colleague Dr Sigmund Freud. Local anaesthetic techniques have many advantages in day surgery and their use is now widespread. In considering these techniques and the drugs, the following headings are used:

- patient preparation
- management during establishment of block
- management during surgery
- management in recovery and of discharge
- local anaesthetic drugs.

It should be noted that the guidelines for management that follow are based on what is considered as best practice by anaesthetists. Many non-anaesthetist users of local anaesthesia (i.e. surgeons) may disagree with some aspects of this routine.

Patient Preparation

The management of patients undergoing an operation under local anaesthesia should be as careful and meticulous as those undergoing general anaesthesia. Anxiety levels may well be high and a considerate approach will yield large dividends. According to Goldman *et al.* (1988), day case surgery is known to elicit anxiety, with many anaesthetists regarding day surgery patients as one of the most anxious groups they have to deal with. They should be pre-assessed and provided with verbal and written information and prepared as much as possible for what they are going to experience. As the maximum dosage of local anaesthetic that may be used is calculated according to the patient's body weight, it is important that this is recorded.

Establishing a rapport with patients can make an important contribution to the success of the technique, perhaps this should be called *vocal anaesthesia.* In an ideal situation patients should be fasted in a similar fashion to that recommended for patients undergoing general anaesthesia (see Chapter 7).

Management During Establishment of the Block

Prior to injection of local anaesthetic most patients should have intravenous access established and be connected to appropriate monitoring. The degree of monitoring used will depend on several factors including:

- fitness of the patient
- size and duration of the proposed procedure and
- quantity of local anaesthesia required.

A fit young person undergoing removal of a small skin lesion may well not require intravenous access or monitoring other than by chatting to them. However, a pulse oximeter takes only seconds to connect to any patient and causes no discomfort, yet it provides useful information to all staff in theatre about the patient's pulse and oxygen saturation. The other extreme may be an elderly person undergoing a cataract extraction; they should have intravenous access established and have pulse oximeter, electrocardiograph (ECG) and blood pressure monitors connected.

Management During Surgery

All patients should have someone to talk and to monitor them throughout the procedure, explaining what is happening when this is necessary but otherwise providing both distraction and encouragement. This may be the anaesthetist if one is involved, but ideally, this should be the circulating nurse. Indeed, establishing a rapport is essential here and provides an important opportunity for theatre staff to develop and use their communication skills.

Management in Recovery and Discharge

Following completion of the procedure, patients may be admitted to recovery or if the procedure has been straightforward and their condition is stable then they may return to the ward area. Management of patients in the ward should be similar to that for patients undergoing general anaesthesia (see later). Patients and their carers should be told what to expect as the local anaesthetic wears off. It is important that local anaesthesia is not used as an excuse to discharge patients quickly with few postoperative instructions and no analgesia. For example, it is not satisfactory practice to quickly discharge vasectomy patients and to tell them to use paracetamol for pain relief.

For larger operations, such as inguinal hernia repair performed under local anaesthesia, it is important that patients are not only provided with analgesics to take home, but also provided with the first dose prior to discharge and *before* the local wears off. Oral analgesics take some time to be absorbed and to provide their effect; it is not good practice therefore to instruct patients to take the first dose when their wound becomes sore.

Local Anaesthetic Drugs

There are three main local anaesthetic drugs in current use – lignocaine, prilocaine and bupivacaine. These agents have differing characteristics that are important for the management of patients. However, their toxic effects are similar and it is important that all staff involved in the management of patients receiving local anaesthesia are aware of them. The signs and symptoms experienced by the patient change as the level of the drug in the blood stream increases; initially the patient may notice a tingling sensation around their mouth, tinnitus or nausea, then the patient will start to feel nervous and if the level continues to rise the patient will lose consciousness or may have a epileptic seizure. Further increases will result in heart dysrhythmias and eventual asystole.

The maximum dose that may be given is calculated on the basis of the patient's weight – for example 2 mg of bupivacaine per kilogram body weight.

The critical level, however, is that achieved in the blood stream (as explained above) by absorption from the site of injection. This rate depends on the blood flow to the area and can be

Learning Points

Signs of local anaesthetic toxicity:

- circumoral tingling
- tinnitus
- nausea/nervousness
- loss of consciousness/seizures
- cardiac dysrhythmias.

Box 8.2 Calculation of maximum dose of local anaesthetic

- **A 1% solution means that 1 g of a substance is dissolved in 100 ml of solvent**
- 1 g is equivalent to 1000 mg. Therefore the concentration per ml is 1000/100 or 10 mg per ml.
- ***Example: dose calculation***
- Patient weighs 70 kg and the surgeon wishes to use 2% lignocaine with no adrenaline.
- ***The maximum dose is 3 mg kg^{-1}*** – therefore dose is 210 mg (70 multiplied by 3)
- 2% lignocaine is equivalent to 20 mg ml $^{-1}$ (i.e. 2 multiplied by 10)
- ***Therefore the surgeon can only use 210 divided by 20 = 10.5 ml.***

reduced for lignocaine and prilocaine by the addition of adrenaline to the local anaesthetic agent. The adrenaline causes local vasoconstriction, thereby reducing the rate of absorption; this also has the beneficial effect of prolonging the block. Therefore, when considering the maximum dose, two figures are quoted: one for the plain local anaesthetic solution and the other for the agent plus adrenaline. One final important point is that these agents are supplied in *percentage solutions*, for example lignocaine 1%. Therefore it is important for staff to understand the conversion of a total dose in milligrams (mg) to millilitres (ml) of the local anaesthetic solution. The easy answer is to remember to multiply the percentage of the solution by 10 and that gives the concentration in mg ml^{-1}. The full explanation for this easy answer is provided in Box 8.2 (for those who are interested in the arithmetic) as is an example of using the calculation.

Lignocaine – maximum dose 3 mg kg^{-1} (plain); 5 mg kg^{-1} (with adrenaline)

Lignocaine is the most commonly used local anaesthetic and was introduced in the late 1940s. Part of its popularity stems from the fact that it has a more rapid onset of action than other available drugs. The local anaesthetic effect lasts a relatively short time – perhaps 90 min when injected with adrenaline.

Prilocaine – maximum dose 5 mg kg^{-1} (plain); 7 mg kg^{-1} (with adrenaline)

Prilocaine has a very low toxicity level as is reflected in the relatively large volumes that can be used. The duration of action is similar to that of lignocaine. It can cause a condition called methaemoglobinaemia in which the patient appears cyanosed. This is not usually a life-threatening problem and interestingly can be treated by the administration of methylene blue intravenously.

Bupivacaine – maximum dose 2 mg kg^{-1} (plain or with adrenaline)

Bupivacaine provides a long duration of action (up to 8 h when used in nerve blocks) which has made it a popular choice for those looking to provide postoperative analgesia. However, it has a slow onset of action – it can take 30 min for a simple nerve block to achieve the full effect. This fact plus the relatively low dose of agent that can be used has limited its appeal to surgeons for infiltration anaesthesia. However, many surgeons now instil or inject bupivacaine into the surgical wound to aid postoperative analgesia during operations performed under general anaesthesia.

General Anaesthesia

Patients in the UK being admitted for an operation expect (on the whole) to be asleep during the procedure. There are interesting differences in this expectation across Europe with the incidence of local anaesthesia being far greater on the continent, and Scandinavia in particular. This may reflect how quickly general anaesthesia became safe in the UK as it was quickly recognized as a medical specialty and attracted many talented doctors.

In this section we examine the following topics:

- terminology and basic techniques in general anaesthesia
- general anaesthetic drugs
- preparation of patients
- management during induction of anaesthesia
- management during surgery
- management in recovery and of discharge.

Terminology and Basic Techniques in General Anaesthesia

General anaesthesia as we have defined on page 114 combines loss of consciousness (hypnosis, sleep) and loss of sensation (analgesia). These form two parts of the *anaesthetic triad*, the third being relaxation. The anaesthetic triad describes the three parts of a general anaesthetic that an anaesthetist has to supply to varying degrees for different operations. For example, during a laparotomy, patients are usually paralysed using a muscle relaxant thus providing maximal relaxation of the abdominal muscles and requiring that patients are ventilated. In contrast, during an arthroscopy, patients are normally allowed to breathe for themselves and only relaxation sufficient to ensure the patient does not move is necessary.

Another term that will be found in anaesthetic texts is *balanced anaesthesia* – this is a term used to describe how anaesthetists achieve the relative amounts of analgesia, relaxation and sleep required by using a combination of relatively small doses of several specific drugs. The advantage of using this technique is that by using smaller doses of several drugs, side-effects associated with the larger doses of a single agent can be avoided. A single anaesthetic agent can provide all three aspects of the triad when given in high enough doses; however, this is associated with high levels of morbidity including nausea and vomiting.

Learning Points

Anaesthetic triad

- analgesia
- relaxation
- hypnosis (sleep)

Balanced anaesthesia

- achievement of above by using small doses of several agents

There are many ways of classifying the type of general anaesthetic being used but fundamentally most anaesthetics can be classified by considering three questions:

- How is the airway is being managed?
- How is the patient is being kept asleep?
- Is the patient breathing for him or herself?

Airway Management

Patient's airways are routinely maintained by one of three choices:

- utilizing a face mask (with or without an airway)
- utilizing the laryngeal mask airway
- utilizing an endotracheal tube (oral or nasal).

In day surgery the laryngeal mask is probably the most common technique used.

Maintenance of Anaesthesia

Patients are kept asleep by the use of:

- inhalational agents
- intravenous infusions of induction agents – total intravenous anaesthesia (TIVA)
- intravenous boli of potent analgesics and major tranquillizers – neuroleptanalgesia.

Neuroleptanalgesia is seldom used in day surgery; inhalational techniques are by far the most common but the use of TIVA is growing.

Mode of Ventilation

Patients may be:

- breathing for themselves – breathing spontaneously
- being ventilated – intermittent positive pressure ventilation.

In day surgery, patients are most commonly allowed to breathe for themselves, but there are procedures for which the anaesthetist may need to paralyse and ventilate the patient. The most common anaesthetic in day surgery is likely to involve the patient breathing spontaneously through a laryngeal mask and being kept asleep by an inhalational agent. Indeed this type of anaesthetic *can* (though not all anaesthetists will) be used for all of the original 20 operations suggested as being suitable for day surgery by the Audit Commission (1990).

General Anaesthetic Drugs

There are many drugs used in general anaesthesia; this section concentrates in providing some information about groups of drugs that will be used in day surgery units. The groups of drugs considered are:

- induction agents
- inhalational agents
- analgesics
- muscle relaxants.

Induction agents

An induction agent is a drug that 'brings on' anaesthesia (i.e. it causes patients to lose consciousness) and the level of this can be altered by adjustment of the dose of the agent. There are many induction agents that may be used in day units, including methohexitone, etomidate and ketamine, but the two that will commonly be seen are *sodium thiopentone* and *propofol*.

Sodium thiopentone

This barbiturate has been the gold standard of induction agents since its introduction in the 1930s. During this period many agents have appeared but have failed to approach the standards set by thiopentone. It has, however, become less popular (for day surgery in particular) with the release of propofol. Induction with thiopentone is rapid, occurring in one arm–brain circulation time which is typically 30–40 s in fit people. It provides a smooth induction with little coughing or patient movement, but in common with all induction agents, it may cause respiratory depression. Patients recover from a single induction dose of thiopentone in a few minutes but this is not due to rapid elimination. Recovery is due to the drug being redistributed from the central nervous system to other tissues in the body (liver and muscle, but mainly fat) and its breakdown and elimination from the body are extremely slow; indeed 30% of the original dose may remain at 24 h.

Propofol

Propofol is one of the more recent anaesthetic agent developments, having been released in the late 1980s. It is supplied as a white emulsion as it is prepared in an intralipid-type preparation not unlike diazemuls. It has a similar rapid onset of action to thiopentone but appears to depress laryngeal reflexes to a greater degree – which may make insertion of the laryngeal mask easier. The speed and quality of recovery of patients who have had propofol is better than thiopentone and indeed it is worthwhile talking to recovery staff who remember its introduction. Attempts to quantify the improvement in journals have not shown the degree of improvement that has been experienced clinically; indeed, many surgeons and recovery nurses have been moved to ask the anaesthetist what they were doing differently when they first started to use propofol! It has a short half-life and is rapidly cleared from the body and this factor has led to its use for maintenance of anaesthesia (TIVA) and its popularity in day surgery.

Inhalation agents

The number of inhalation agents that may be seen in day units is rapidly increasing; however, those that are most common are nitrous oxide, halothane, enflurane and isoflurane. There are several new agents (*sevoflurane and desflurane*) that will be seen in some units but the position these agents will hold is not yet known and will depend on their cost and any advantages perceived by the anaesthetists that use them.

Nitrous oxide

Ths is more commonly known as laughing gas and is used in anaesthesia and in the provision of analgesia by paramedics at accidents, by nursing staff on burns wards and by midwives on delivery units in the form of entonox. It provides excellent analgesia which is of rapid onset (20–30 s), continuing whilst the patient remains breathing it, but wearing off quickly when discontinued. These characteristics explain its popularity in trauma, pregnancy and burns units. It is not possible to anaesthetise a patient with nitrous oxide alone but it provides a useful part of most anaesthetists balanced anaesthesia technique. The other inhalational agents are also known as *volatile* agents and are the main agents used to keep patients anaesthetized. The term 'volatile' in this context is not the term used to describe a surgeon who regularly throws instruments about the theatre! Rather, it describes the ability of liquid agents to evaporate at room temperature.

Halothane

This was introduced in the 1950s and still offers some advantages over the more modern agents. It does not have the nasty smell of the other agents which makes it more pleasant for patients to breathe – this is especially important where the anaesthetist wishes to use a gaseous induction, for example with children. Unfortunately, it has been linked to causing a severe hepatitis in some patients and although this risk is extremely low, it has reduced its use. It should not be given more frequently than 6 monthly.

Enflurane

This was introduced in the 1960s and as a development of ether has a strong smell that is irritant to patients. This disadvantage is compounded by the fact that it is less potent than halothane and so larger concentrations have to be given. It should not be used in patients with a history of epilepsy.

Isoflurane

This was introduced in the 1980s and is an isomer of enflurane; that is, the same components but put together slightly differently. It therefore also has an irritant smell but is more potent than enflurane. It can be used safely in epileptic patients. Its characteristics produce more rapid recovery from anaesthesia than either halothane or enflurane.

Relaxants

Muscle relaxants are used in anaesthesia to paralyse the patient either as part of the balanced anaesthetic technique, for example to allow the surgeon access to the abdomen, or to enable the anaesthetist to intubate the patient to protect the airway, for example when the surgeon is removing wisdom teeth. There are two main groups of muscle relaxants in common use:

- depolarizing muscle relaxants
- non-depolarizing muscle relaxants.

Depolarizing muscle relaxants

Suxamethonium is the only commonly used drug of this type. It acts by mimicking acetylcholine at the neuromuscular junction so as it attaches to the receptor it causes the muscle to depolarize – this causes the muscle movement (fasciculations) seen with this drug. A large percentage of patients experience severe muscular pains for some days following its administration. These tend to be worse in young patients who ambulate quickly, therefore many day units attempt to avoid its use. One of the reasons for its continued use by anaesthetists is that it provides excellent intubating conditions very quickly (30–60 s) and only lasts for about 5 min. Prolonged paralysis for several hours can occur (scoline apnoea) in patients with a low or atypical form of the plasma enzyme pseudocholinesterase. This complication, however, is extremely rare.

Non-depolarizing muscle relaxants

This is a much larger group of drugs, examples of which include atracurium, mivacurium and vecuronium. Each of these drugs has its own pharmacological profile but we consider this group as a whole. They all act by competing with acetylcholine for the receptors at the neuromuscular junction. They have a slower onset of action than suxamethonium and their duration of action is longer, varying from 10 to 30 min. They do not cause problems with muscular pains following their use and unlike suxamethonium they can be *reversed* by the use of anticholinesterases such as neostigmine.

Analgesics

The analgesic drugs commonly used intra-operatively by anaesthetists include fentanyl, alfentanyl, morphine and papaveretum (Semple & Jackson 1991). Generally, in day surgery practice the longer-acting opioids, morphine and papaveretum (omnopon) are used much less.

Fentanyl

Fentanyl was introduced in the 1960s and is a relatively short-acting opioid analgesic. Its duration of effect depends on the dosage given, but typically is around 20–30 min.

Alfentanyl

This drug was introduced in the 1980s and has two characteristics that make it interesting to anaesthetists. First, it has a very rapid onset of action. Most analgesics including fentanyl take several minutes to achieve their maximum effect whilst alfentanyl takes less than 2 min. Second, it has a very short duration of action; that is about 10 min.

Both these agents are used extensively in day surgery anaesthesia because of their short duration of action. This aids the fast recovery of patients from their anaesthetic. However, their short duration will also lead to the faster return of pain unless something else is done. Therefore, there is still a role that can be played by the older agents with a longer duration of action.

Morphine and papaveretum

These are the oldest analgesics known to man and are obtained from the opium poppy (*Paper somniferum*). They take up to 20 min to reach their peak effect and provide analgesia for about 4 h. Nausea and vomiting are a problem after these agents particularly in ambulant patients, so requiring careful use in day surgery practice.

Non-steroidal anti-inflammatory agents (NSAIDs)

These drugs are commonly used in day surgery as they offer the advantage of providing analgesia with little or no incidence of nausea, vomiting, dependence and respiratory depression. However, when used alone they do not provide sufficient analgesia for many operations, therefore they are commonly used in combination with the opioids. Using them in this manner reduces the need for opiates by as much as 20% (Cashman 1993). Until recently Voltarol was not available for intravenous use and had to be given orally, intramuscularly or by suppository. Following problems surrounding consent for the insertion of suppositories in anaesthetized patients it is important that units have guidelines for their use. Care must also be taken when giving this drug intramuscularly as it can be painful for the patient. Ketorolac is available as an intravenous or intramuscular injection and for oral intake.

Certain groups of patients should not be given these agents including patients with a history of:

- peptic ulceration
- allergy to aspirin
- moderate or severe renal failure.

Problems can also occur in asthmatic patients but if the patient has used aspirin or one of the commercially available NSAIDs with no problems then they can and should be considered (Frew 1994).

Patient Preparation

Patients undergoing day surgery are usually unpremedicated and therefore anxiety levels may be high (Goldman *et al.* 1988, Markland & Hardy 1993). Anxious patients that are unprepared and ill-informed are more difficult to anaesthetize as they tend to require larger doses of induction agents and develop problems such as coughing and laryngospasm. Therefore, patient preparation is important. This should start with the pre-admission assessment process dealt with in Chapter 5. Pre-admission assessment has many functions but should include:

- screening function
- answering patients queries
- provision of written and verbal information about both operation and anaesthetic.

It is important to provide the anaesthetic perspective on the need for screening day surgery patients. It should be obvious already from this chapter that the health of patients may have an effect on the anaesthetic that will be used, for example if a patient is epileptic, the anaesthetist will avoid enflurane. The anaesthetist will be interested in a history of:

- epilepsy
- diabetes
- hypertension
- heart disease
- obesity
- blood problems, e.g. sickle cell anaemia
- muscle disease
- previous anaesthetic problems – patient or family
- current drugs
- allergies.

No categorical recommendations can be made about what a pre-admission assessment system should contain but it should now be obvious that involvement of the anaesthetic department in setting up the system is essential to ensure that patients are selected appropriately. Failure to involve the anaesthetic department will result in the risk of patients being cancelled on the day of surgery despite having passed through the pre-admission assessment system. There is one further topic that requires discussion with the anaesthetic department and should be covered with each patient who attends for pre-admission assessment and that is *fasting*. As discussed in Chapter 7, tradition has dictated that patients who are to undergo a general anaesthetic be fasted for 4–6 h prior to theatre. A more rational period of fasting for both adults and children is now being adopted (Strunin 1993, Phillips *et al.* 1994) and an example of such a new guideline is:

- no solids to eat within 4 h of surgery
- drink normally until within 4 h of surgery
- allow up to $\frac{1}{2}$ pint (275 ml) of fluid – juice, tea or coffee up to within 2 h of surgery.

Patient preparation does not end at pre-admission assessment and the reception and support of patients on the day of admission plays a vital role (see Chapter 7). During this phase patients should receive a visit from their anaesthetist so they have the opportunity to discuss their anaesthetic. At this pre-operative review the anaesthetist will be interested in patients':

- weight
- blood pressure
- current medication
- allergies
- past medical, surgical and anaesthetic history
- smoking habits
- dentition.

This visit should provide reassurance for patients and the chance for the anaesthetist to discuss any special anaesthetic technique that is planned. In particular, patients should be warned about the use of local anaesthetic techniques and consent obtained for the insertion of any suppositories (e.g. Voltarol). It is recommended that all staff read the recent articles about this subject (e.g. Mitchell *et al.* 1995).

Management During Induction of Anaesthesia

> Although the environment in which anaesthesia is administered is usually a carefully controlled area, the anaesthetic agents and the patient's response to them can be unpredictable. (Wilson 1995)

All patients should be accompanied to the anaesthetic room by the nurse looking after them in the ward area. It is essential that nurses establish a rapport with the patients in their care, especially those who are anxious. Holding the patient's hand is common practice, but tone of voice, gestures and facial expression can all be used to convey an empathic presence and support (Kneedler & Dodge 1991). Nurses should always remain in the anaesthetic room until patients are asleep. The anaesthetist will establish intravenous access and the necessary monitoring (see later). Anaesthesia is then induced and the airway secured. Following successful induction, and only when the anaesthetist is happy to proceed, should patients be taken into theatre.

Management During Surgery

Once patients are anaesthetized they are totally dependent on the anaesthetist and all theatre staff for their physical well-being. This not only includes the obvious management of the anaesthetic by the anaesthetist but also includes moving patients from trolley to operating table and the care during positioning (for more detailed discussion, see Chapter 9). Monitoring of the patient is vital to provide safe anaesthesia and several national and international recommendations have been published about minimal standards of monitoring of patients under general anaesthesia (Association of Anaesthetists 1988, International Task Force On Safety In Anaesthesia 1993). The degree of monitoring necessary alters according to the type of anaesthetic being given and the type and size of operation. The typical day unit theatre should provide:

- ECG
- pulse oximetry
- non-invasive blood pressure monitor
- capnography
- temperature monitor.

Specific care and management in recovery is discussed in full in Chapter 10.

Analgesia Following Day Surgery

This aspect of patient care is pivotal to the success and popularity of day surgery. Such is the attention on this facet of care today that it is difficult to imagine that the problem of unsatisfactory pain control following surgery was largely ignored in this country up to the end of the 1980s. In 1990, a report was published from a joint working party of the Royal College of Surgeons and the then College of Anaesthetists called 'Pain after Surgery'. This was a landmark publication and is well worth the effort to find and read (see recommended reading at the end of the chapter).

Having just started to get the management of pain high on the agenda for inpatients, it is essential that the large numbers of patients now being transferred to day surgery do not suffer at home. Although as professionals we are sure this would not be allowed to happen, such poor

Figure 8.1 Prescription form for children

Oral Analgesia Prescription for Children

Day Surgery and Treatment Unit

Patient label

Weight ....kg
Consultant Surgeon ....

Dose: The dose of codeine phosphate (orally) is 0.5 mg kg^{-1} 4 hourly, maximum of 5 doses in 24 h. It is supplied as codeine phospate syrup 25 mg 5 ml^{-1}. For ease of administration the dose should be rounded up or down to the nearest 0.5 ml.
Please countersign the prescription for the dose indicated as appropriate for this child.

Weight range	Dosage prescribed	Signature
7.5–12.5 kg	1.0 ml (5 mg) 4 hourly	....
12.6–17.5 kg	1.5 ml (7.5 mg) 4 hourly	....
17.6–22.5 kg	2.0 ml (10 mg) 4 hourly	....
22.6–27.5 kg	2.5 ml (12.5 mg) 4 hourly	....
27.6–32.5 kg	3.0 ml (15 mg) 4 hourly	....
32.6–37.5 kg	3.5 ml (17.5 mg) 4 hourly	....
37.6–42.5 kg	4.0 ml (20 mg) 4 hourly	....

Dispensed by .... Checked by ....

practice would quickly reduce the popularity of day surgery with patients and their general practitioners.

The first stage of successful pain control occurs in the theatre, as we have already discussed, with the use of local anaesthesia and of intra-operative analgesics. The next stage is ensuring that patients are comfortable at each stage of their recovery and before they are discharged from the unit. The use of pain-scoring systems such as linear analogue scales or verbal rating systems is recommended and a good review of the methods available to measure pain and their limitations can be found in Carroll and Bowsher (1993).

Although all pain theories and models tell us that only the individual suffering is able to define their pain, both medical and nursing staff still tend to underestimate the degree of pain and discomfort experienced by patients following surgery. Some procedures are perceived by professionals as relatively painless, for example hysteroscopy, dilatation and curretage, vasectomy and insertion of grommets. However, experience shows us that a large proportion of patients undergoing such procedures frequently suffer a great deal of pain and simple analgesics such as paracetamol are clearly not effective. However, this is not the only problem. A large number of patients have low expectations of pain control; that is, they expect to suffer following surgery. Hume *et al.* (1994) studied the knowledge of anaesthesia and peri-operative care of 166 patients undergoing gynaecological, urological and general surgical procedures. Forty-eight per cent of patients thought pain to be a part of healing and 39% saw pain as something to be endured. It is

Figure 8.2 Prescription form for adults

Oral Analgesia Prescription for Adults

Day Surgery and Treatment Unit

Patient label | Consultant

Please prescribe oral analgesia for patients on this form. Four choices are provided for analgesia depending on expected severity of discomfort following the operation. Non-standard analgesia regimes may still be prescribed on the patient's discharge letter on the few occasions this should be necessary. Each patient will receive one standard dayunit pack of the drugs prescribed.

Minor

Drug	**Dosage**	**Signature**
Co-codamol 8/500	2 tablets 4–6 hourly	....

Intermediate

Drug	**Dosage**	**Signature**
Diclofenac (Voltarol)	50 mg 8 hourly	
Codydramol	1–2 tablets 4–6 hourly	....

Major

Drug	**Dosage**	**Signature**
Diclofenac (Voltarol)	50 mg 8 hourly	
Co-codamol 30/500	1–2 capsules 4–6 hourly	....

Prescription where there is contraindication to non-steroidal drugs

Intermediate or Major

Drug	**Dosage**	**Signature**
Co-codamol 30/500	1–2 capsules 4–6 hourly	

Dispensed by.. **Checked by** ....

not surprising, therefore, that compliance with prescribed analgesia is often poor. But these problems respond to education – both of clinicians and patients.

There are several ways of improving the prescribing of analgesics by clinicians responsible for patients. The use of separate prescribing charts for children (Fig. 8.1) and adults (Fig. 8.2) that require a single signature is important to ensure that the prescription of analgesics is as easy as possible. This allows us to move to a more rational and consistent approach to analgesia prescription.

Operations are linked into groups according to the severity of the postoperative pain experienced by patients. These are graded in severity as in Table 8.1 where prescriptions exist for mild, moderate and severe pain groups. It is only through audit of our current practice and these developments that we can ensure that patients receive the care they deserve (see

Table 8.1 Operative related groups for analgesia

Mild
Myringotomy
Hysteroscopy

Moderate
Vasectomy
Loop excision of transformation zone of cervix (cone biopsy)
Carpal tunnel surgery
Cystoscopy
Termination of pregnancy

Severe
Arthroscopy
Kellers osteotomy or other bunion surgery
Dupuytren's contracture surgery
Laparoscopic sterilization
Wisdom teeth extraction
Hernia repair
Varicose vein surgery

Chapter 12). However, acceptance and compassion remain the central ingredients of any analgesia protocol (Burden 1993).

Analgesics Used Following Day Surgery

Most analgesics used following day surgery are based on paracetamol, codeine or dihydrocodeine and the NSAIDs. Paracetamol alone is of little use for the postoperative pain of most procedures. Though it has formed the mainstay of analgesia following paediatric surgery, there is evidence that it is insufficient following many procedures (Mather & Mackie 1983). In paediatric practice we need a liquid preparation of any drug and there are two main drugs that may be used:

- ibuprofen
- codeine phosphate.

Ibuprofen

This is an NSAID and in the paediatric elixir form is indicated for the control of mild to moderate pain. It is not recommended for children under 1 year of age. The same care is required as for the prescribing of NSAIDs in adults (see page 124).

Codeine phosphate

This is available as an elixir that may be used in children of all ages, but it should be remembered that codeine phosphate can cause constipation.

Some recent American research has been exploring the possibility of *fentanyl* lollipops! Although there would clearly be difficulties in regulating the distribution of the drug throughout the lollipop, and controlling the dosage, as Burden (1993) points out, the most worrying aspect is the explicit linking of drugs with sweets.

With adults, there is a far larger choice of agents that can be used. Although most of these are combinations of paracetamol with codeine or dihydrocodeine, there are other drugs available, such as paracetamol in combination with a drug called dextropropoxyphene. This latter agent, though popular in the past, has considerable problems with side-effects and the potential development of dependence and should be avoided.

Summary

In this chapter we have covered the differences between anaesthesia, sedation and local anaesthesia. The management of the patient throughout their visit has been explored from an anaesthetic point of view and the management of their pain both peri-operatively and postoperatively considered. This chapter is designed to provide a baseline knowledge of anaesthesia and analgesia in day surgery. It is hoped that the reader will take this baseline and consider the practice in their own unit and help move the management of day surgery patients forward.

Key Points

- General anaesthesia was first successfully used in 1846.
- Local anaesthesia was first successfully used 20 years later.
- Sedation is a technique in which the use of a drug or drugs produces a state of depression of the central nervous system enabling treatment to be carried out, but during which verbal contact with the patient is maintained.
- General anaesthesia is any technique in which a drug or combination of drugs produces loss of sensation and loss of consciousness, as defined by failure to respond to verbal command.
- Sedation techniques have considerable inherent dangers and patients undergoing sedation should be monitored and given supplemental oxygen.
- Sedo-analgesic techniques increase the risk of respiratory depression.

Recommended Reading

The Royal College of Surgeons of England & The College of Anaesthetists (1990) **Pain after surgery: Report of a working party of the commission on the provision of surgical services.** The Royal College of Surgeons of England and The College of Anaesthetists.

Wilson, J. (1995) **Clinical risk management. Building provider awareness in the administration of anaesthesia.** *British Journal of Theatre Nursing* **4**(12): 8–11

This article is based on a case study involving high-risk practice and introduces the principles of risk management. It is well worth reading

Whitwam, J. G. (Ed) (1994) **Day Case Anaesthesia & Sedation**. Oxford: Blackwell Scientific Publications

An excellent readable text covering a range of topics pertinent to day-case anaesthesia

References

Association of Anaesthetists of Great Britain and Ireland (1988) **Recommendations on standards of monitoring.** Association of Anaesthetists of Great Britain and Ireland.

Audit Commission (1990) **A short cut to better services: Day surgery in England and Wales**. London: HMSO.

Bell, G. D., McCloy, R. F., Charlton, J. E., Campbell, D., Dent, N. A., Gear, M. L. W., Logan, L. F. A. and Swan, C. H. J. (1991) **Recommendations for standards of sedation and patient monitoring during gastrointestinal endoscopy.** *GUT* **32**: 823–827.

Burden, N. (1993) **Ambulatory Surgery Nursing**. Philadelphia: Saunders.

Carroll, D. and Bowsher, D. (1993) **Pain: Management and Nursing Care**. London: Butterworth–Heinemann.

Cashman, J. N. (1993) **Non-steroidal anti-inflammatory drugs versus post-operative pain.** *Journal of the Royal Society of Medicine* **86**: 464–467.

Charlton, J. E. (1995) **Monitoring and supplemental oxygen during endoscopy: One death per 2000 procedures demands action.** *British Medical Journal* **310**: 886–887.

Coplans, M. P. and Curson, I. (1982) **Deaths associated with dentistry.** *British Dental Journal* **153**: 357–362.

Frew, A. (1994) **Selected side-effects: 13. Non-steroidal anti-inflammatory drugs and asthma.** *Prescribers' Journal* **34**: 74–77.

Goldmann, L., Ogg, T. W. and Levey, A. B. (1988) **Hypnosis and day-case anaesthesia.** *Anaesthesia* **42**: 466–469.

Hume, M. A., Kennedy, B. and Ashbury, A. J. (1994) **Patient knowledge of anaesthesia and perioperative care.** *Anaesthesia* **49**: 715–718.

Kneedler, J. A. and Dodge, G. H. (1991) **Perioperative Patient Care** (Second Edition). Boston: Jones & Bartlett.

Markland, D. and Hardy, L. (1993) **Anxiety, relaxation and anaesthesia for day-case surgery.** *British Journal of Clinical Psychology* **32**: 493–504.

Mather, L. and Mackie, J. (1983) **The incidence of post-operative pain in children.** *Pain* **15**: 271–282.

Mitchell, J. (1995) **Fundamental problem of consent.** *British Medical Journal* **370**: 43.

Phillips, S., Daborn, A. K. and Hatch, D. J. (1994) **Preoperative fasting for paediatric anaesthesia.** *British Journal of Anaesthesia* **73**: 529–536.

Poswillo, D. E. (1990) **General anaesthesia, sedation and resuscitation in dentistry: Report of an expert working party.**

Semple, P. and Jackson, I. (1991) **Postoperative pain control – a survey of current practice.** *Anaesthesia* **46**: 1074–1076.

Strunin, L. (1993) **How long should patients fast before surgery? Time for new guidelines.** *British Journal of Anaesthesia* **70**: 1–3.

International Task Force On Safety In Anaesthesia (1993) **The International Task Force On Safety In Anaesthesia.** *European Journal of Anaesthesiology* **10**: Supplement 7.

The Royal College of Anaesthetists & The Royal College of Radiologists (1992) **Report of a joint working party on sedation and anaesthesia in radiology.**

Wilson, J. (1995) **Clinical risk management. Building provider awareness in the administration of anaesthesia.** *British Journal of Theatre Nursing* **4**(12): 8–11.

Wylie Report (1981) **Report of the working party on training in dental anaesthesia.** *British Dental Journal* **151**: 385–388.

Chapter 9 Key issues in theatre practice and clinical management

Overview

This chapter is concerned primarily with the team work, understanding and collaboration necessary in the theatre area to maintain the level of safe practice that is in the best interests of patients and staff. The fast throughput of patients in day theatres creates a real potential for error that demands diligent personnel and active management. Adopting a risk assessment and management approach and concentrating upon the vital contribution of key personnel, the fundamental requirements of communication, co-operation and mutual understanding are explored.

Chapter Focus

- Developing a clinical risk management strategy
- Principles of safety and common risk occurrence areas
- Communication
- Infection control
- Control of the environment
- Care of equipment
- Moving, positioning and manual handling
- Nursing roles and functions collaborative working

Introduction

Patients undergoing surgical procedures are dependent totally on the theatre team for their safety and well-being. In an 'average' theatre, patients are exposed to anaesthetic agents, chemicals, electricity and radiation in addition to a degree of physical and psychological trauma. Orem (1991) identifies the 'prevention of hazards' as one of *seven universal self-care needs* (see Chapter 6) and as such, patients have the right to protection and remain free from harm; this is the responsibility of all theatre personnel. The team comprises (in no particular order of importance):

- anaesthetist
- surgeon
- scrubbed assistant
- circulator
- operating department assistant (if utilized in your Trust).

The team relies on the support of:

- ward staff
- portering services
- pharmacy
- physiotherapy
- radiography
- medical records staff.

The provision of a safe environment is clearly dependent on good teamwork; the success of which depends to a large extent on all team members readiness to understand, respect and support the role and responsibilities of the other members. This can sometimes be lacking with potentially serious consequences.

Clinical Risk Management

However roles and functions are defined, the prime concern for all theatre personnel is the maintenance of a safe environment for patients and staff.

Risk management is concerned with identifying and measuring risks with the ultimate purpose of reducing the frequency of adverse events and harm to patients to the benefit of patient care. It should not be exercised as a reactive 'witch hunt', solely organized to root out unsafe practitioners. Neither is it about disciplinary action, 'covering up' or encouraging defensive practice (Clements 1995). All staff must be able to claim ownership of the strategy and see their role in it. According to Wilson (1995a), clinical risk management (CRM) co-ordinates methods of assessing risk with quality standards and relevant legislation and is defined as:

> The systematic identification, assessment and reduction of risks to patients and staff and the prevention and avoidance of untoward incidences and events (Wilson 1995a).

CRM is therefore proactive, focusing on risks to patients, staff and business (Simpson 1995). A CRM strategy typically involves three essential elements as shown in Box 9.1.

Although we are introducing the concept of risk management in the context of theatre, it should be evident that assessment of risk covers *all* aspects of the patient experience of day surgery, from pre-admission assessment to discharge. The success of any risk-management programme hinges on the following factors:

- *Continuity of care* – the fewer different people involved in a patient's care, the less the margin is for error (as identified in Chapter 7).
- *Leadership and supervision* – it goes almost without saying that inadequate supervision of staff and anaesthetized patients is one of the most commonly identified causes of error – 'Unconscious patients in theatre rarely cause their own injuries' (Wilson 1995a).
- *Staff with appropriate skills and levels of competence* – again this seems self-explanatory, but making the right appointments based on sound skill mix review and analysis of need will always be the best way to proceed.
- *Adequate staffing levels* – essential for safe practice.

Box 9.1 A clinical risk management strategy (Wilson 1995a)

1. Awareness and evaluation

- assessing the present situation
- identifying potential and actual risk areas
- taking this message to those areas (Clements 1995)
- documenting this fully – unfortunately, some risk management programmes stop at this stage; the strategy needs to move beyond mere assessment.

2. Education and implementation

- assigning responsibility for specific areas; to include ways of avoiding or minimizing that risk
- allowing staff to identify 'trigger events' in their own area
- encouraging all staff to assess own practices that could contribute to placing patients at risk (Wilson 1995b)
- looking for ways to track trends of occurrences.

3. Integration and support

- establishing a means of reporting incidents in which staff are not blamed or professionally isolated
- investigating when appropriate.

- *Effective communications strategy* – effective written and verbal communication underpins all safe practice.
- *Accurate, factual documentation of events* – remember all documents are legal documents in a court of law (see Chapter 7).

In day theatre areas with a fast throughput of patients, it is not difficult to identify potential risk-occurrence areas; some may sound ridiculous, but these events do happen, for example:

- absence of medical notes
- the wrong patient, therefore the wrong operation
- right patient but wrong operation
- brakes not applied to trolley
- incorrect drug or drug dose given
- patient allergies not noted
- incorrect swab/instrument count
- doubtful or questionable consent
- patient falls off table
- tourniquets left on too long.

Learning Points

Clinical risk management comprises three main elements:

- awareness and evaluation
- implementation and education
- integration and support.

General Safeguards

Communication

The literature repeatedly identifies effective communication as the most important safeguard available to all personnel (Lewis 1994, Simpson 1995, Wilson 1995a,b). Communication in this instance means verbal and written, and 'effective' refers to both content and means. All communications must be clear and unambiguous. The use of jargon and abbreviations should be avoided to prevent misinterpretation by staff unfamiliar with the language. All patients should be referred to by name, not 'the first case' or 'the next patient' (Medical Defence Union *et al.* 1986). All care and management must be documented fully and legibly by the individuals concerned and *all* must be signed (see section on legal aspects of record keeping in Chapter 6). Care plans should be completed in a uniform way across all theatres to protect patients and staff and must be seen as an integral part of care (UKCC 1993).

Skills in assertiveness are essential to all nurses. The seemingly easy going and friendly relationships that are developed within the theatre team can both facilitate and militate against open communication. Much depends on the ground rules established when the team comes together; unfortunately, these rules are part of the theatre culture and are rarely openly discussed, yet are quite tangible.

Sadly still accepted, sexist forms of communication within the team may similarly prevent nurses from reporting a potential error for fear of damaging a relationship that has taken time to develop. But nurses cannot truly say they are the patient's advocate if this kind of behaviour and communication repeatedly goes unchallenged and this again underlines the importance of individual accountability for practice.

It appears that there is little specific guidance from professional bodies to help theatre nurses deal with this apparently widespread problem. However, until more nurses accept that the potential damage to both their patients and their profession is more important than special relationships, the position is unlikely to change.

That said, all staff must respond immediately and appropriately in the event of an error (Burden 1993). It is also worthwhile to consider clause 2 of the UKCC Code of Professional Conduct;

> Ensure that no action or omission on your part or within your sphere of responsibility, is detrimental to the interests, condition or safety of patients and clients. (UKCC 1992)

Reflection Points

It appears to be acceptable for surgeons to say whatever they like, in whatever language they like, to whomever they choose, regardless of how offensive or unprofessional it might be. These comments can be directed at patients or members of staff.

- Have you had to deal with this kind of situation?
- If so, what action did you take?
- How did taking that action make you feel?
- Do nurses more frequently rely on non-verbal messages (especially eye movements witnessed over the top of the mask) to communicate their dissatisfaction with a comment?
- Do they challenge either content or style of delivery?
- If not, why might this be?

A very specific communication issue concerns instrument, swab and needle counts; established and universally understood protocols are essential (Wilson 1995a). Day surgery procedures are often quite short, but repetitive and pressure to 'get on' with the list and other distractions must not be allowed to interfere with this vital safety check that hinges on clear verbal and written communication. Possible sources of error in maintaining accurate counts include excessive haemorrhage and failure to count swabs in superficial operations (Medical Defence Union *et al.* 1986). Wilson (1995a) also makes the point that even though surgeons have overall responsibility and delegate instrument and swab counting, nursing staff may still be found liable if those counts are incorrect.

Infection Control

General Measures

A large number of issues can be explored under this broad heading that indicates the importance of infection-control measures in reducing risk occurrences. Clearly, the maintenance of asepsis is vital during surgery. It requires continuous awareness and responsibility of those in theatre for their actions and the potential risks of those actions. General principles for control of infection should include:

- ensuring general health and standards of hygiene of theatre personnel are appropriate for the job they are doing (difficult to deal with but essential) – all skin lesions, sore throats and diarrhoea should be reported (Pediani 1993)
- limiting access to theatre to authorized and appropriately clothed personnel; i.e. reviewing *who* is wearing *what* and *where*
- changing clothing when soiled
- changing masks frequently with careful handling (Pediani 1993); 'wearing a used mask around the neck is somewhat akin to wearing a used handkerchief around the neck' (Burden 1993)
- female staff wearing trousers instead of traditional theatre dresses
- using only sterile equipment and instruments and always checking expiry dates
- adopting a rational approach to theatre cleaning; e.g. as dedicated theatres will not have been used overnight, it is best to keep air movement and early morning activity to a minimum, therefore 'energetic' damp dusting is not appropriate (Mackrodt 1994)
- using appropriate, effective and rational scrub, gowning and gloving techniques
- disposing of waste/body fluids/tissue promptly in an accepted manner in line with local infection control guidelines and policies
- being alert to possible needlestick or scalpel injury, especially scrubbed personnel.

Universal Precautions

These are the safe practices designed to protect both patients and staff from blood-borne infection; the principle behind this concept being that 'blood and certain body fluids of all patients must be considered potentially infectious for blood borne pathogens' (Taylor 1993). The simple fact is that even the best clinicians and state of the art technology cannot reliably identify all those infected with human immunodeficiency virus (HIV) or hepatitis B virus (HBV). Taylor

(1993) argues that it is no longer acceptable to label certain patients as 'high risk' on account of their lifestyle, sexual preferences or medical history and such practice can lead to a false sense of security when caring for 'non or low' risk patients. Universal precautions require that all patients' blood and body fluids are treated in the same manner and the handling of such is kept to a minimum (Burden 1993). Such changes will require a substantial and ongoing investment in both time and money and will not be implemented overnight. However, as Taylor and Quick (1994) point out, the adoption of universal precautions and concentration on blood-borne infections can lead to other micro-organisms transmitted through routes other than blood, such as methicillin resistant *Staphylococcus aureus* (MRSA), being ignored. No hospital can afford to do that.

Control of the Environment

Day surgery units are not the same as main theatre complexes. Shared rest rooms for ward and theatre staff and the everyday movement of different groups of staff and patients from 'public' to theatre areas that is so much a part of day surgery could also be placing patients at risk. These activities and practices need to be closely monitored and, if necessary, restricted in some way. Burden (1993) points out that a balance must be achieved between creating a comfortable and less-threatening environment for day surgery patients and the potential for occurrence of infection.

Theatres and anaesthetic rooms must have effective air change systems and appropriate anaesthetic gas scavenging. In common with recovery areas (see next chapter), temperature and humidity need to be maintained within set parameters. Keeping theatre doors closed at all times and controlling staff movement in and out of theatres helps prevent air contamination and maintains the necessary ventilation (Pediani 1993). Also beware of trailing cables and flexes on theatre floors.

Care of Equipment

It is beyond the scope of this text to examine the different instruments and their specific uses in surgical procedures; the reader is advised to consult one of the two texts specifically highlighted at the end of the chapter. However, it is important to appreciate some of the general principles of inspecting instruments prior to and following surgery in order to minimize injury to patients. West (1992) suggests the following are checked:

- all instrument components present and working
- joints of instruments operate smoothly
- ratchet fastenings grip in all settings
- points of all types of forceps are in alignment
- scissors are sharp
- insulation intact on diathermy instruments.

Diathermy

All staff using diathermy equipment must have a basic understanding of how it works, the effects on body tissue, the hazards associated with its use and appropriate safeguards (Kneedler & Dodge 1991, West 1992). Manufacturers' instructions must be followed. It is vital that the patient electrode makes good contact and spirit-based disinfectants are allowed to evaporate prior to use of diathermy (Medical Defence Union *et al.* 1986). Any malfunctioning equipment must be immediately removed from use, labelled to that effect and reported in the appropriate manner. Any equipment or instrument that the nurse is unhappy with or uncertain about should not be used.

Lasers

Theatre personnel need to understand and adhere to guidelines regarding use of laser equipment; it is essential that local policies and protocols are accessible and updated (Frost 1993). The laser is rapidly becoming an accepted surgical tool; their tissue vaporization effect causes minimal thermal damage to surrounding tissues. Eye protection should be worn by awake patients and personnel in theatre and warning signs should be placed on the doors into theatre (Kneedler & Dodge 1991).

Maintenance and repairs of all equipment should be documented, signed and dated. Updating on new equipment for all relevant staff is essential before it is put into use (Wilson 1995a). Similarly, adherence to the regulations governing the Control of Substances Hazardous to Health (COSHH) is essential, particularly in relation to the widespread use of glutaraldehyde (Hutt 1994), for staff and patient safety.

Manual Handling/Patient Positioning

The movement and positioning of unconscious patients requires planning, co-ordination and care. All members of the theatre team have individual and collective responsibility for patient well-being (Wilson 1995a). Patients should not be moved without the anaesthetist's agreement and then slowly and gently to avoid injury. Burden (1993) states that proper positioning ensures correct anatomical alignment and avoids circulatory or nerve impairment; there should be no pressure on bony prominences or nerves and little on skin; 'it is interesting to note the number of studies indicating intra-operative injuries that look like burns and are reported as burns, but are actually the result of pressure' (Burden 1993). Box 9.2 outlines the action to safeguard against intra-operative patient injury; much of the responsibility for ensuring these actions are taken rests with the circulating nurse and the scrubbed assistant at the table. Pressure points must be protected during surgery and checked at the end of the procedure to ensure no damage has occurred (West 1992).

Box 9.2 Preventing injury to patients during surgery (adapted from Burden 1993)

- Ensure arms are not hyperextended past 90° to prevent brachial plexus injury
- Ensure no body parts extend over edge of operating table or trolley
- Ensure unprotected body parts are not touching metal or unpadded surfaces
- Ensure patients' legs in supine position remain uncrossed
- Place pillow between patients' legs when in lateral position
- Ensure patients' legs are moved into lithotomy poles simultaneously by two people
- Use a patient-moving device, such as *Patslide* or *Easislide*; **never** pull or push an unconscious patient
- Ensure no team member either leans on or places heavy instruments on a patient

Haigh (1993) points out that all theatre personnel are required to act in accordance with the EEC directive on manual handling operations (EEC 1990) and section 7 of the Health & Safety at Work Act 1974 (HMSO 1974). These demand that staff:

- avoid the need for hazardous manual handling operations
- assess any hazardous operations that cannot be avoided
- take action to remove/reduce risk of injury based on that assessment
- make full and proper use of any relevant equipment.

Safety protocols and policies are established to protect patients and staff from the numerous hazards associated with working in an operating theatre. As errors largely occur as a result of a breakdown in communication and short cuts in care delivery taken in the interests of speed, understanding and collaboration between staff is essential.

Nursing Roles and Functions and Collaborative Working

Nurses in day theatres appear to be experiencing the same kinds of difficulties in defining their role and function as their colleagues in inpatient theatre areas. In hospitals that employ operating department assistants (ODAs) and furthermore, support and fund their education, nurses are defining their role and preparing to defend it against all comers.

Unfortunately, this issue is clouded by the fact that many qualified nurses still involve themselves in what Webb (1995) describes as a 'myriad of non-nursing, task-orientated activities'. She suggests that such activities frequently include:

- restocking prep rooms with supplies
- ordering and putting away stores
- answering telephones and pagers
- acting as a messenger for surgeons and anaesthetists
- fetching and carrying non-urgent equipment
- damp dusting and preparing theatre furniture before lists
- clearing away equipment and cleaning between cases and at the end of each list.

There are probably a lot more, and none of these tasks requires 3 years pre-registration nurse education to accomplish. In our experience, an 8-week 'theatre' placement as a student nurse, albeit some years ago, actually involved 8 weeks of plastic bag folding, shelf tidying and trolley wheel cleaning, with very little patient contact. We suggest that patients and their individual needs are at risk of 'getting lost' as nurses seek to define and justify their role in theatres. It almost seems that nurses, feeling threatened by ODAs' technical expertise and good relationships

Reflection Point

In this present climate of skill mix and value for money, are senior experienced nurses in theatre simply an expensive luxury? What are the reasons for continuing to employ nurses in theatre areas? Are these reasons justifiable?

(For further discussion, see page 142)

with anaesthetists, are attempting to cordon off the surgeons and the technology that goes along with the specialty. (It is interesting that despite having undergone training and education in anaesthetics, theatre and recovery, ODAs are to be found almost exclusively in the anaesthetic rooms.)

> Theatre nurses have almost disappeared behind operating theatre barriers, becoming so engulfed with machinery and gadgetry that they have lost track of the patient. (Leonard & Kalideen 1985)

As surgery becomes even more 'high-tech', this position is likely to continue, unless tackled in a rational manner. Greater understanding at a national level (BJTN 1994) is not necessarily translating into improved relationships in individual theatres. Furthermore, continued professional 'jealousy' can prevent both groups from looking at how they can collaborate in the interests of safety and quality of care for patients.

Pre-operative Visiting

One of the ways that theatre nurses have responded to questions about what they actually do is to be found in the quite abundant literature on pre-operative visiting. Although this literature is grounded in main theatre areas, it is worthy of some discussion as the limits of the practice are evident. Much of the interest and subsequent largely anecdotal and non-research-based accounts appear to be based on one piece of work – that of Lindeman and Stetzer in the USA, published in 1973. This research examined the effects of a pre-operative visit from a theatre nurse on the experiences of 176 surgical patients. The study's findings suggest that theatre and recovery nursing care are enhanced because the staff have more information about patients and that post-operative anxiety were reduced in those who were visited. A more recent study (Martin 1996) also suggests that anxiety is significantly reduced. The beneficial effects of state anxiety discussed in Chapter 7 were not addressed by either study, nor were the effects of teaching cognitive coping strategies or relaxation; anxiety is simply defined as undesirable and information is the answer. The latter study also suffers from a small and unrepresentative sample, unmatched groups and some rather sweeping suggestions for future practice.

Although both these studies have clearly identified one possible facet of theatre nurses' role, neither have explicitly recognized that (a) only those patients who seek information will benefit from planned procedural information, and (b) it is more likely that the improved information brought about the reduction in anxiety, *not* who provided it.

Another important issue in this debate concerns the communication skills of the theatre nurses involved in pre-operative visiting. A pre-operative visit should have clear objectives in terms of patient outcome; it is not just a social chat. As clearly outlined in Chapter 4, there is considerable evidence that suggests that both the quality and quantity of nurse–patient interaction is poor. If direct interaction with patients has not been a principal feature of theatre nurses' role, McKay (1995) is right to caution against embarking on pre-operative visiting.

For those who are determined to demonstrate the need for theatre nurses to undertake this role, research needs to compare the effects of the same information on patient experiences when provided by a visiting theatre nurse and the ward nurse. Perhaps energy would be better expended in improving theatre and ward liaison and facilitating perioperative care (i.e. total nursing care during anaesthesia, surgery and recovery) within the theatre complex.

Reflection Points

With greater freedom of movement between ward and theatre, nurses in day surgery units are in the ideal position to facilitate perioperative care.

- Do nurses in theatres routinely visit patients pre-operatively in your day surgery unit?
- If so,can you identify the organizational and management factors that are supporting the practice?
- If it is not happening, what are the principal barriers to change?

Is Day Surgery Different?

Anecdotal evidence suggests that day surgery units have appeal as they offer varied experience and more opportunities for theatre nurses to form relationships with patients, however short term. After all, most people become nurses because they want to be with and care for people. Whilst it would be fair to say that, in an integrated unit, theatre nurses are in an ideal position to visit patients both pre- and postoperatively (i.e. become more involved), apparently still very few choose to do so. Both surgeons and anaesthetists generally visit their patients prior to and following surgery, yet both nurses and ODAs appear content to 'care' for total strangers.

Greater collaboration with primarily ward-based nursing staff can reap huge benefits for both patient and staff satisfaction. There is no reason why theatre- and recovery-based nurses cannot or should not be primary nurses. However, whilst theatre nurses continue to perform non-nursing activities, the cry of 'we haven't got time to do all that' (i.e. get more involved in patient care), will continue to be heard. More worrying is the belief of some theatre nurses that they are not employed to do that. Unfortunately, this attitude begs the question that if theatre nurses are not involved with patient care, why are they employed in theatres at all? This is a question that a lot of Trusts are asking. Furthermore, anecdotal evidence suggests that patients are often quite surprised to find that nurses work in theatres. The *scrubbed* and *circulating* roles of nurses in theatres are the principal roles, but they are obviously not visible to patients. The ways in which these roles and their associated responsibilities are often defined (e.g. West 1992) further question the need for nurses in theatre. McGee (1994) cites the views of some nurses that a 'trained monkey' could scrub and pass instruments during an operation. Whilst not suggesting that we employ some friendly primates to work in theatres, there is room for greater flexibility and utilization of different personnel.

Principal Nursing Roles in Theatres

Registered nurses in theatres are normally engaged in one of two distinct roles, the circulating role and the scrubbed role. The 'circulator' (a bad term) or 'runner' (worse) are both terms that seriously underplay the importance of this role in any theatre. West (1992) is rather guilty of this when she describes the circulator as 'the nurse or operating department assistant who helps the scrubbed assistant to prepare for the operation'. Some of the circulator's responsibilities before, during and after surgery are set out in Box 9.3.

Box 9.3 Examples of circulator's responsibilities (taken from West 1992)

Before the operation:

- checks theatre has been cleaned and equipment is working
- collects necessary equipment
- prepares gowns and gloves for the team and assists in tying gowns
- opens instrument packs and bowls.

During the operation:

- remains in theatre throughout
- connects diathermy and suction leads
- adheres to local policy for swab disposal
- fills bowls with sterile water
- records blood loss
- assists with swab counts.

After the operation:

- helps with removal of drapes
- removes instrument trolley to dirty utility area
- ensures theatre is cleaned and prepared for next case.

At no time is any responsibility to the patient made explicit – so defined, it is easy to question if this is a nursing role and West is right to suggest that it could be undertaken by other personnel. Health care assistants can be taught to tie surgeons' gowns, open packs, pour water into bowls and count swabs. With time and training anyone can learn surgeons' different preferences, anticipate the need for extra instruments and the use of the many different types of suture material. But we would argue that the circulating and support role *is* best carried out by nurses, but only when it is explicitly recognized that their principal responsibility is to patients, not simply the scrubbed team. Patients undergoing general anaesthesia are dependent on theatre personnel and nurses in particular for their care whilst in this vulnerable position. If we think back to Orem's (1991) three nursing systems (see Chapter 6), nursing in this context is clearly *wholly compensatory* – that is, patients have no active role in their care; nurses need to both do for and act for patients. Nursing as defined by Orem involves:

- doing or acting for another (includes the role of patient advocate)
- guiding and directing for another (providing information)
- providing physical support (a partnership)
- providing psychological support (empathic presence)
- providing an environment which supports development
- teaching.

The skills required to fulfil this patient-centred role are arguably more important and certainly need to be made more explicit; essential skills therefore include:

- observation – of patients condition, potential and actual hazards and threats to patient well-being and safety
- anticipation of patients and colleagues needs
- highly developed communication skills, both verbal and written
- understanding of potential responses to anxiety and fear, therefore enabling appropriate and individually tailored physical and emotional support for patients undergoing procedures under local anaesthesia and sedation
- assertiveness skills to speak and act in patients' interests
- protection of patients' dignity and privacy
- accurate documentation of intra-operative patient care
- close liaison with ward and recovery staff.

This is a role that centres on safety and well-being of patients and is underpinned by professional responsibility and accountability. Clearly, nurses are and should be able to provide assistance for the surgical team, thereby contributing to safe practice but as McGee (1994) puts it, 'only as part of learning to fulfil the true nursing role'.

Likewise, fulfilling the *scrubbed* role requires dexterity and skill in anticipation and observation with expertise borne out of plentiful practice. It requires total concentration and is fast becoming more and more technical in nature. Such skills are clearly worth developing but they should not become the sole reason for nurses being in theatres. Whilst recognizing these skills and vital safety aspects associated with fulfilling this role, it could just as easily be carried out by appropriately trained ODAs. They are well qualified and are equally able to anticipate and plan ahead (Jackson 1993). The scrubbed assistant role is defined by West (1992) as 'the member of staff who prepares the sterilised instruments and equipment ready for the operation'. Again, there is no implicit or explicit recognition of nursing function in this definition. In 1966, Virginia Henderson offered this now famous definition of nursing:

> The unique function of the nurse is to assist the individual sick or well in the performance of those activities . . . that he (she) would do unaided if he (she) had the necessary strength, will or knowledge. And to do this in such a way as to help him (her) gain independence as rapidly as possible. (Henderson 1966)

Placing the tongue firmly in cheek, translated into the role of the scrubbed assistant this becomes:

> The unique function of the scrub nurse is to assist the surgeon, good or ill tempered, in the performance of those activities that he or she is well capable of doing unaided if only he or she had the necessary strength, will or knowledge. And to do so in such a way that the surgeon's role as superior being is reinforced and the *status quo* maintained

We concur with Kneedler and Dodge (1991) and argue that it is the circulating role that is the key nurse's role in a theatre area, *not* the scrub role, yet it is this that is ascribed superior status. However, this 'superior' role often involves quite senior nurses running round during their 'break' preparing refreshments for the surgeon and anaesthetist. Roberts (1989) and Kneedler and Dodge (1991) believe that 'scrubbing' is held in much higher regard by theatre nurses than those activities which generally involve being with patients who are awake. As McGee (1994) points out, 'the surgeon, the anaesthetist, the scrub nurse and the assistant make an exclusive team'. Being a

Reflection Points

- Why do you think theatre nurses value the scrubbed role so highly?
- Is it a *nursing* role? If so, why? If not, why not?

member of this team is bound to provide job satisfaction and a feeling of equality with consultants that perhaps ward nurses cannot achieve. It must go a long way to explain the continued fascination with the job, but it cannot truly be called nursing as regardless of the knowledge, dexterity and skills involved, the needs of the surgical team clearly assume priority over those of patients.

Other theatre personnel, especially students, remain rather on the outside, excluded from this team which along with the 'tea ceremonies', is the principal reason for students' dissatisfaction with theatre placements. Indeed, so few were the opportunities to learn about patient care, that pre-registration nurse education (UKCC 1986) no longer requires that students undertake a theatre placement. McGee (1994) argues that 'there is something seriously wrong if students cannot see theatre nursing as centring around the patient'. But this appears to be the case for both pre- and postregistration students, with the latter group often finding it even more difficult to understand and accept such 'elitism' and lack of inclusion or support from their peer group. The focus of nursing practice in theatres is illness; therefore, some conflict is bound to arise between current understanding of what nursing is and what theatre nurses actually do. There is little doubt that recruitment to theatre areas at present is ineffective but it is by no means certain that this situation can be partly or wholly attributed to falling student placements.

Theatre nurses, even more than ward nurses, use a non-patient-centred language. Half an hour in the staff room reveals frequent references to 'lists', 'the first case', 'gasmen', 'locals', 'majors and minors', 'STOPs' or 'colps'; not patients, care plans or nursing care. This tendency to follow a procedure-centred (as opposed to patient-centred) model of practice and theatre nurses' apparent reluctance to document nursing care only serves to reinforce the view that nursing does not actually take place in an operating theatre after all (Lewis 1994).

Theatre Nursing in Day Surgery

Day surgery units seem to offer more opportunity to break down some of the traditional barriers, to renegotiate roles and functions and work more in collaboration with ODAs in the provision of total patient care. This current ideal – the peri-operative role – is quite easily achievable in day surgery units, but its development relies heavily on vision, strong and effective leadership and a climate of trust in which all staff feel able to openly discuss both their aspirations and fears. Given our understanding of patients needs, Box 9.4 underlines the major reasons why nurses are needed in day theatre.

All of the functions described in Box 9.4 assume even greater clarity and importance when viewed in the context of day surgery. In addition, they are best achieved when nurses are *not* permanently tethered to an operating table and when effective management and leadership promotes safe flexible practice and personal and professional growth.

Box 9.4 Why nurses are needed in theatres (adapted from Webb 1995)

- To reinforce preparatory information and provide support for patients before, during and after surgical procedures that are performed under a local anaesthetic
- To provide support and information before and after surgical procedures that are performed under a general anaesthetic
- To act as patients' advocate, maintaining patient dignity and privacy
- To teach – patients (pre-operatively), student nurses, trainee ODAs, colleagues and new nursing staff
- To manage lists and provide support for theatre teams
- To liaise with ward and recovery staff to ensure consistent and individualized care
- To evaluate care through audit and selective postoperative visiting

Specific Clinical Management Issues in Day Theatres

Operating Lists

Effective management in theatres is essential for the safety and well-being of patients and staff and this clearly involves the management and control of individual operating lists (Evans 1991). A major problem is the emphasis on reducing waiting lists and achieving set thresholds and this will drive the numbers on a given list. All it takes is an error of judgement in estimating the number who will fail to attend to result in far too many patients on one operating list. Not wanting to cancel any operations, this pressure is transferred on to theatre staff to 'get through' the list as soon as possible in order to free space for afternoon lists. Not surprisingly, breaks then assume low priority, when in fact they should be enforced. It is often assumed that 10 short cases must be less stressful for the scrubbed team than a couple of major ones. However, the onset of fatigue and failing attention is closely associated with automatic, non-critical performance with an increased likelihood of potentially disastrous errors.

In order for facilities to remain efficient, operating sessions must be used appropriately with surgeons providing adequate notice for non-utilization of lists. Whilst it is no bad thing for all staff to appreciate the costs involved, as Jackson (1993) points out, it is unfair to expect staff to take unutilized theatre time as time owed or annual leave. Although this practice solves a problem in the short term, it will do little for morale and the retention of valued and experienced staff.

Educational Needs of Staff

Experienced and motivated theatre nurses who are keen to raise standards of nursing practice and teach others are in quite short supply (Jackson 1993). A rational educational programme must be established, based on skills assessment and needs analysis. In day surgery units especially, considerable opportunities exist for nurses to extend their repertoire of clinically relevant skills and develop a perioperative approach to patient management. Access to the National Vocational Qualification (NVQ) in Operating Department Practice at level 3 is one option available that can improve flexibility and utilization of staff (Havill & Walker 1994). Likewise, established courses in day surgery (ENB A21 & N33) actively promote a perioperative approach. Utilization of individual development review (IDR) for all grades of nursing staff helps to match individual skills, educational needs and objectives for personal and professional development with the developing needs of the service. It may be desirable, for example, for some nurses to undertake a course specifically in day surgery and others in theatre practice (ENB 176). In addition, supporting some individuals on a critical care course (ENB 100) will broaden experience and repertoire of skills in anaesthetic and recovery skills for core nursing staff. Managers must be prepared to review the necessary mix of skills and support the appointment of appropriate ancillary support staff within the unit to assume responsibility for non-nursing tasks. Only then will theatre nurses be able to do what they are there to do: care for patients.

Summary

The safety and well-being of patients during day surgery procedures is paramount and depends on collaboration, diligence and support. The theatre complex is a potentially hazardous environment that requires effective leadership and a rigorous programme of risk assessment and management, in the interests of both patients and staff. It is likely that the debate surrounding nurses in theatres will continue for years to come; developments such as nurse surgical assistants are receiving close attention and may be seen by some as a way of strengthening nurses' position in theatres. The personal and professional ramifications of such roles are discussed more fully in Chapter 13. However, at the very least, a system of ongoing IDR and educational needs analysis is essential in order to retain valued and experienced staff.

Key Points

- Day theatres have a fast throughput which increases the potential for mistakes; working under pressure increases fatigue, encourages automatic non-critical performance and compromises patient safety.
- Effective leadership and management is essential.
- Teamwork, support and continuity of care is vital in maintaining patient safety.
- Clinical risk management applies to all aspects of the day surgery experience and is concerned with protecting patients from injury or harm.
- Safety protocols must be rational and evidence based.
- Effective verbal and written communication underpins safe practice.
- Greater staff flexibility is dependent on letting go of traditional ideas about nursing roles in theatres; ODAs are well able to undertake the scrub role.
- Nurses *are* needed in theatres, but their vital role in patient care, teaching and support must be made more explicit and attention given to assessment, planning, implementation, evaluation and documentation of care; greater development of the *perioperative role* would achieve this.

Recommended Reading

Kneedler, J. A. and Dodge, G. H. (1991) **Perioperative Patient Care** (Second Edition). Boston: Jones & Bartlett

This text includes particularly clear and useful chapters on instruments and equipment, maintenance of asepsis, patient positioning, performing counts and documenting patient care (Chapters 20–24 inclusive). Although some of the instruments names vary (the text is American), the chapters are readable and very comprehensive

National Association of Theatre Nurses (1994) **Principles of safe practice in the operating theatre**. Harrogate: NATN

An excellent resource for safety information although somewhat expensive; every unit should have access to a reference copy

West, B. J. M. (1992) **Theatre Nursing: Technique and Care** (Sixth Edition). London: Baillière Tindall

Simple, cheap and easy to read, this text includes useful information and photographic material in the areas of infection control, surgical instrumentation and hazards in theatre

References

BJTN (editorial) (1994) **Working together.** *British Journal of Theatre Nursing* **4**(1): 19–21.

Burden, N. (1993) **Ambulatory Surgical Nursing**. Philadelphia: W. B. Saunders.

Clements, R. V. (1995) **Essentials of clinical risk management.** *Quality in Health Care* **4**: 129–134.

EEC (1990) **Council directive on the minimum handling of loads.** *Official Journal of the European Community* No L 156/9.

Evans, E. (1991) **Nurses in the operating theatre.** *Surgical Nurse* **4**(1): 10–15.

Frost, J. (1993) **Clinical application of lasers.** *Professional Nurse* **8**(5): 298–303.

Haigh, C. (1993) **Manual Handling – a review of the new legislation.** *British Journal of Theatre Nursing* March 93, 4–6.

Hatfield, A. and Tronson, M. (1992) **The Complete Recovery Room Book**. Oxford: OUP.

Havill, C. and Walker, J. (1994) **Working together – national vocational qualification in operating department practice.** *Surgical Nurse* **7**(4): 9–13.

Henderson, V. (1996) **The Nature of Nursing: a Definition and its Implications for Practice, Reseach and Education.** New York: Macmillan.

HMSO (1974) **Health & Safety at Work Act**. London: HMSO.

Hutt, G. (1994) **Glutaraldehyde revisited.** *British Journal of Theatre Nursing* **3**(10): 10–11.

Jackson, A. (1993) **Theatre issues – a manager's viewpoint.** *Surgical Nurse* **6**(4): 11–14.

Kneedler, J. A. and Dodge, G. H. (1991) **Perioperative Patient Care** (Second Edition). Boston: Jones & Bartlett.

Leonard, M. D. and Kalideen, D. (1985) **So, you're going to have an operation.** *NAT News*; February, 12–21.

Lewis, M. (1994) **Communication in theatres.** *Surgical Nurse* **7**(1): 27–29.

Lindeman, C. A. and Stetzer, S. L. (1973) **Effect of preoperative visits by operating room nurses.** *Nursing Research* **22**(1): 4–16.

Mackrodt, K. (1994) **Damp dusting in the operating theatre: implications for bacteria counts.** *British Journal of Theatre Nursing* **4**(9): 10–13.

Martin, D. (1996) **Pre-operative visits to reduce patient anxiety: a study.** *Nursing Standard* **10**(23): 33–38.

McGee, P. (1994) **Rediscovering theatre nursing.** *British Journal of Theatre Nursing* **4**(3): 8–10.

McKay, K. (1995) **Is theatre nursing 'nursing'?** Unpublished BA Thesis, University of Manchester.

Medical Defence Union (1993) **Theatre safeguards, consent, anaesthetic risks and day unit surgery.** London. MDU.

Medical Defence Union *et al.* (1986) **Theatre Safeguards.** London: MDU.

NATN (1994) **Principles of safe practice in the operating theatre.** Harrogate: NATN.

Orem, D. E. (1991) **Nursing: Concepts of Practice** (Fourth Edition). New York: McGraw-Hill.

Pediani, R. (1993) **Hazards and safety in theatre.** *British Journal of Theatre Nursing* March 93, 19–21.

Roberts, S. (1989) **Going, going, gone: theatre nursing.** *Nursing Times* **85**(40): 61–65.

Simpson, A. (1995) **A framework for identifying and managing risk in the operating theatre.** *British Journal of Theatre Nursing* **5**(6): 5–8.

Taylor, M. (1993) **Universal precautions in the operating department.** *British Journal of Theatre Nursing* January 93, 4–7.

Taylor, M. and Quick, A. (1994) **MRSA in the operating department.** *British Journal of Theatre Nursing* **3**(10): 4–7.

UKCC (1986) **A New Preparation for Practice (Project 2000).** London: UKCC.

UKCC (1992) **Code of Professional Conduct.** London: UKCC.

UKCC (1993) **Standards for Records and Record Keeping.** London: UKCC.

Unerman, E. (1994) **Infection control in the operating department.** *Surgical Nurse* **7**(1): 31–34.

Webb, R. A. (1995) **Preoperative visiting from the perspective of the theatre nurse.** *British Journal of Nursing* **4**(16): 919–925.

West, B. J. M. (1992) **Theatre Nursing: Technique and Care** (Sixth Edition). London: Baillière Tindall.

Wilson, J. (1995a) **Clinical risk management in theatres. Professional practice: Are you a team player?** *British Journal of Theatre Nursing* **4**(11): 5–7.

Wilson, J. (1995b) **Clinical risk management. Building provider awareness in the administration of anaesthesia.** *British Journal of Theatre Nursing* **4**(12): 8–11.

Chapter 10 Management of first-stage recovery

Overview

This chapter introduces the facilities and skills that are necessary for nurses to provide a safe recovery for patients following day surgery. Recovery requirements for patients undergoing procedures under sedation, local anaesthesia and general anaesthesia are explored and the design of a suitable recovery area and how it should be equipped is discussed. The care of patients in the recovery area and the management of emergencies are considered to help the reader reflect on their practice, experience and future learning needs.

Chapter Focus

- Provision of recovery facilities with regards to structure, situation, equipment and staffing
- Physical and psychological management of patients in first-stage recovery
- Assessment of recovery
- Management of recovery room emergencies

Introduction

In this chapter we consider the initial recovery period of the patient, known as first-stage recovery. (Second-stage recovery is considered in the subsequent chapter.) It is perhaps worthwhile to review the development of recovery areas in theatres over the past decade. To do so, it is necessary to consider the following issues:

- legal responsibility and accountability for the care of patients recovering from anaesthesia
- the need for a rational approach to care
- the development of recovery areas adjacent to theatres.

First and foremost, *the anaesthetist caring for a patient continues to be responsible for that patient until they have recovered sufficiently to be returned to the ward.* Guidelines published by the Association of Anaesthetists (Working Party Report 1985) stipulate that:

> if the anaesthetist is personally unable to remain with the patient during the recovery period he/she should satisfy theirself that the patient is transferred to the care of nursing staff who have been *specially trained in recovery techniques* and have the *expertise* and the *facilities* to manage possible complications.

Furthermore, the anaesthetist:

> should ensure that the nurse is satisfied with the condition of the patient and that he/she knows where to find them should an emergency arise. If they are not going to be available theirself, they should make arrangements for a *medically-qualified deputy* who can oversee the care of their patient.

Whilst this seems to answer the question about responsibility, it does not make explicit the issue of accountability. A more recent report from the Association of Anaesthetists (Immediate Postanaesthetic Recovery 1993) recognizes the need for clarity in terms of accountability. This excellent report is available from the Association of Anaesthetists and is recommended reading for all personnel working in this field. It states that:

> if the anaesthetist is unable to remain with the patient during their recovery, accountability for the patient's care must be transferred to staff who have been specially trained in recovery procedures.

Recovery areas have been developed as a consequence of recognizing the responsibility of the anaesthetist for the recovering patient. If each anaesthetist was to stay with their patients until they had recovered sufficiently to return to the ward, then the number of patients that could be managed on a theatre list would be drastically reduced! Alternatively, more than one anaesthetist would be required to manage each list but with a resultant increase in costs. However, even with two anaesthetists it would only take one patient with a prolonged recovery time to upset the session and lead to cancellations. A further problem would lie with the imperative to recover patients quickly within this system. This could lead to patients being returned to the ward before their cardiovascular system is stable and their postoperative analgesia had been optimized.

The vital role of the nurse in recovery therefore becomes clear as does the location of recovery areas adjacent to theatres. Whilst the anaesthetist remains responsible for the patient, but transfers this responsibility to an appropriately trained nurse, it is vital that they remain able to respond *quickly* should difficulties develop. Nurses must be able to contact the anaesthetist immediately if there is a problem. This is the fundamental reason for the development of recovery areas as part of theatre complexes as only in this situation can a rapid response be assured. A further important point is that this position ensures that unconscious patients are not being transferred long distances between theatres and the recovery area.

Learning Points

- Responsibility for the well-being of the patient recovering from anaesthesia remains with the anaesthetist until the patient can be returned to the ward safely.
- Accountability transfers to the staff in recovery.
- Patients can be transferred to the care of appropriately trained nursing staff who have both the expertise and the facilities to manage possible complications.
- Before transferring care, the anaesthetist should ensure that the nurse is satisfied with the condition of the patient, the postoperative instructions and of their availability should a problem arise.

Structure and Equipment

Recovery Room

A recovery area comprises of a series of bays that provide all the services required for recovering patients. The number of bays required varies with the number of theatres and endoscopy rooms, the type of surgery undertaken and the type of anaesthesia or sedation used. A general guide is that 1.5 bays are required per theatre (Farman 1978) but more may be necessary with rapid turnover as in day surgery (Hudson 1979) or indeed with the rapid turnover but slower recovery that follows sedation for endoscopy. Recommended floor space for a standard bay is 9.3 m^2 with additional room for movement of trolleys and personnel (Utting 1984). Further recommendations include (DHSS 1983):

- room temperature maintained close to 21–22°C
- relative humidity of 38–45%
- minimum of 15 air changes per hour.

The provision of sufficient electric and telephone sockets, sinks and clinical waste services is important. However, more vital is the supply of oxygen and suction. Each bay should be equipped with piped oxygen and vacuum outlets.

Oxygen

This outlet should have the necessary flowmeter and tubing to supply oxygen to recovering patients. There should be a choice of attachments to the oxygen tubing to cater for the recovery requirements of patients and for administrating 100% in an emergency. Thus, a suitable oxygen mask, T-piece attachment and anaesthetic circuit or self-inflating bag and mask should be immediately available to the nurse responsible for the patient. Figure 10.1 shows a suitable set-up for both oxygen and suction.

Figure 10.1 Oxygen and suction supply with suitable attachments

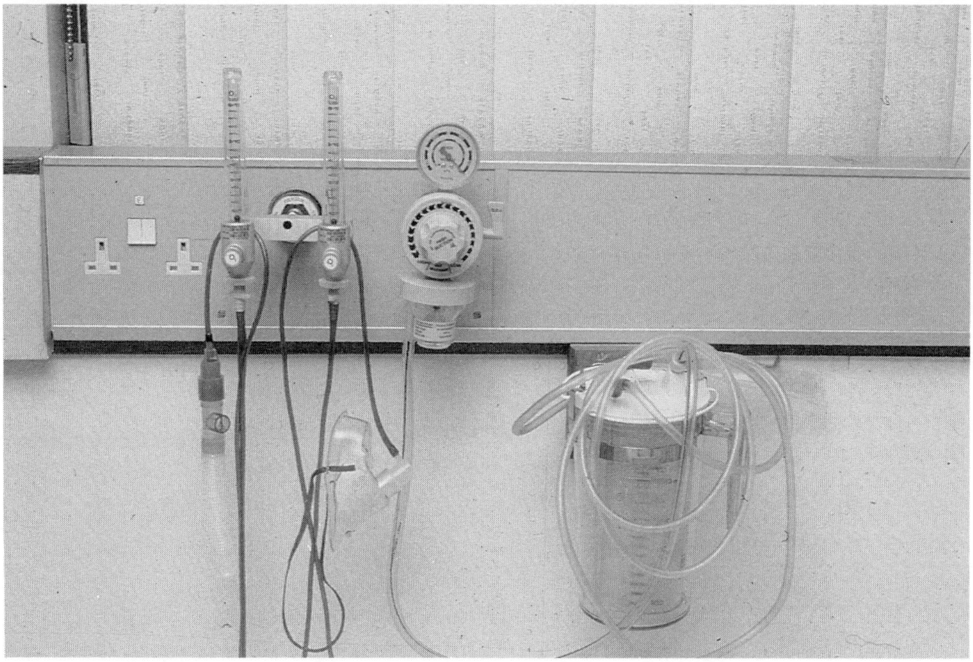

Suction

Again, this outlet should have the necessary suction control and reservoir connected and ready to use. This apparatus should be of a high vacuum type capable of aspirating 35 $l\,min^{-1}$ so that it can deal quickly with vomitus which may endanger the airway (Ward 1985). Suction tubing and a Yankaeur sucker should be attached and replaced if used before the next patient. Suction catheters suitable for endotracheal suction should be available within easy reach.

Additional Equipment

Each bay should also be equipped with a:

- sharps disposal box
- store of swabs, adhesive tape, syringes, needles and canulae
- range of oropharyngeal and nasopharyngeal airways
- suitable container for contaminated re-usable equipment
- supply of vomit bowls and tissues
- suitably sized waste bin.

Clearly, for nurses to provide undivided attention to patients it is important that this equipment is within reach (Figure 10.2). One further vital piece of equipment is a method of calling for assistance. This may be as simple as a referee's whistle or attack-type alarm worn by nurses or maybe a more sophisticated call alarm linked into individual theatres. Whichever is

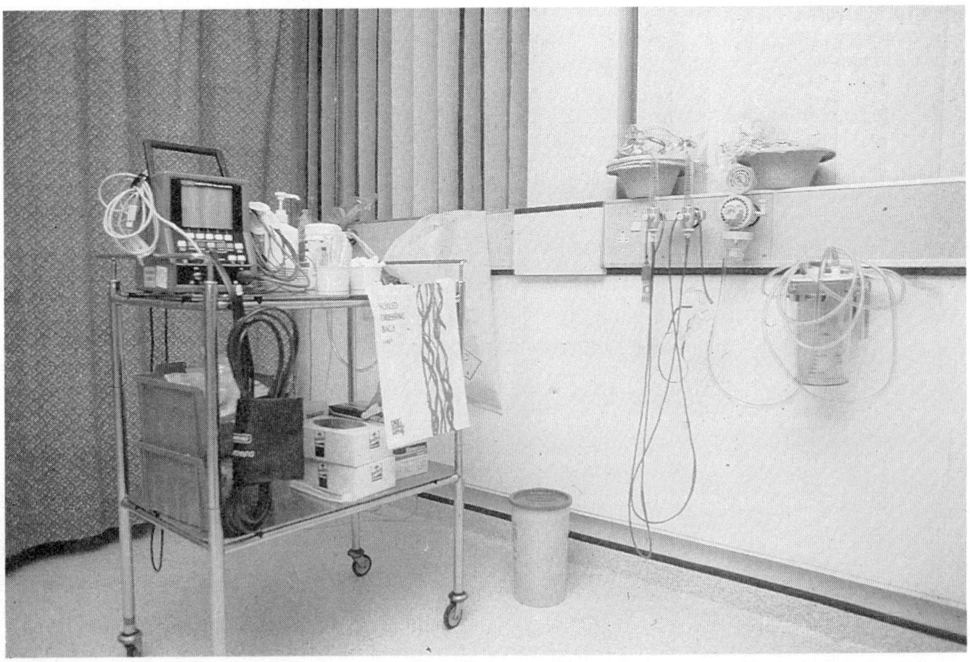

Figure 10.2 Example of a day unit recovery bay

used, it is vital that the signal is *clearly* understood by all users of the theatre complex. The following sections give some further comprehensive guidance for necessary equipment for the safe management of first stage recovery.

Monitoring

Each recovery bay should be equipped with a:

- pulse oximeter
- electrocardiograph (ECG) monitor
- automatic blood pressure monitor or a sphygmomanometer and stethoscope.

General Equipment Shared Within the Recovery Area

Paediatric Equipment

If paediatric day surgery is undertaken in the unit it is advisable to set up a special trolley with the appropriate equipment for recovering children. This should include:

- paediatric blood pressure cuffs and pulse oximeter probes
- paediatric airways, laryngoscopes, endotracheal tubes and breathing circuit
- paediatric resuscitation equipment.

Cardiorespiratory Support Equipment

- primary airway management equipment – airways, laryngeal masks, endotracheal tubes, introducers, gum elastic bougies and laryngoscopes
- primary venous access equipment – selection of canulae and infusion sets
- defibrillator – preferably integrated ECG monitor defibrillator with recorder
- secondary airway management equipment – cricothyroid puncture set and a pre-assembled oxygen supply T-piece set
- nebulizing equipment and masks suitable for the administration of nebulized drugs such as salbutamol.

Miscellaneous Equipment

- thermometer
- peripheral nerve stimulator
- blood sugar measuring equipment (BM stix, dextrostix)
- clearly visible clock with second hand
- refrigerator for drug storage
- storage for intravenous fluids.

In addition, all recovery areas also require a stock of drugs and storage facilities for routine, resuscitation and controlled drugs.

Drugs

The unit should maintain the necessary cardiac arrest drugs and have them easily accessible, preferably with the defibrillator. There are certain drugs that may be needed quickly or more frequently that are suitable to organize for each recovery bay or on a shared basis. These include:

- atropine
- naloxone
- doxapram
- an antiemetic
- reversal agent – neostigmine and glycopyrronium.

Further drugs that should be available include those suitable for the treatment of anaphylaxis and access to a supply of dantrolene for the treatment of malignant hyperpyrexia.

Trolleys

Having given some consideration to the overall design and necessary equipment in a recovery area, there is one further important piece of equipment that we must consider – the patient trolley. In day surgery, the majority of patients will enter recovery on a trolley. The design of this often forgotten piece of equipment is vital to the safe management of patients throughout their stay in the unit. A trolley should have certain key features

- ability to rapidly tilt the patient head down (Trendelenburg tilt) – this must be easily applied by a single person from the head of the trolley
- sides of an adequate length and height to keep the patient on the trolley
- availability of cushioned sides for infants and children
- adjustable backrest support
- comfortable mattress (this is vital in day surgery where the patient will remain on the trolley)
- the wheels should be lockable
- the trolley and mattress should be easy to clean.

The desirability of other features, such as the ability to attach arm boards and lithotomy poles, will depend on whether the trolley is also used as the operating table. Trolleys designed for multipurpose use are now being produced and are proving to be popular but costly. Some trolleys have inherent problems and any unit should fully evaluate those available prior to purchase of this expensive item.

Staffing

We have already identified that staff working in a recovery area need to be specially trained in recovery procedures. According to Drain (1994), nursing staff that are 'well educated, highly skilled and flexible' are the most important ingredient in a successful recovery area. Nurses need to be effective communicators, able to form and maintain sound working relationships with other team members. A clear and expressed commitment to patient comfort and quality of care is every bit as important as knowledge of more technological aspects of recovery care. Most importantly, nurses in recovery must be able to make decisions based on sound clinical judgement and initiate action. In a day surgery unit, recovery is the area to which most staff rotate in order to gain skills and understanding. However, the recovery area must be managed effectively and a core staff deployed there, who then take responsibility for the training of others. As many staff receive their training in this manner, it is important that the content is consistent and should include:

- understanding of the relevant anatomy, physiology and pharmacology
- understanding and experience of the management of the airway in anaesthetized patients
- understanding of monitoring requirements and of the equipment used
- training in resuscitation and the management of emergencies
- understanding of the needs of patients, parents and relatives.

Staff should be formally assessed to an agreed standard. The recently introduced National Vocational Qualification (NVQ) in Operating Department Practice (level 3) provides a useful opportunity for developing local training (for more information regarding this qualification see recommended reading at the end of this chapter). Specific and relevant postregistration nursing courses such as anaesthetic nursing (ENB 182), theatre nursing (ENB 176) and day surgery nursing (ENB A21) provide invaluable experience and increase the flexibility of staff.

The number of staff required will depend on the number of bays that will be used. In the initial recovery period the patient requires 'continuous individual observation on a one-to-one basis and during this period the staff cannot have any other duties' (Association of Anaesthetists 1993). Therefore, it is necessary to staff recovery at a level suitable to maintain both safe, quality care and the throughput from the theatres. It is also important that nurses are not pressurized into managing more than one unconscious patient each. If this position is reached then either the anaesthetist should remain with their patient or more trained staff found.

Management of the Recovery Period

Prelist Check List

Before the start of each day it is vital that nursing staff check all equipment and drugs in their area. This should be formalized with a checklist that is followed and signed each day. The checklist should include:

- ensuring that oxygen supply and delivery systems (breathing circuits) are functioning
- ensuring that the suction is clean and functioning
- ensuring that monitoring equipment is functioning
- ensuring that airway equipment and laryngoscopes are functioning
- ensuring that re-breathe bags are intact
- ensuring that the appropriate drugs are available and within their expiry date
- ensuring that emergency alarms function
- resuscitation equipment including drugs and defibrillator should also be checked on an agreed frequency.

Patient Management

Given the critical care type environments that recovery areas clearly are and the many requirements to ensure safe and uncomplicated recovery, it is perhaps too easy to concentrate on the physiological and technological aspects of nursing management at the expense of the caring role. However, as Drain (1994) points out, assessment of patients' psychological and emotional well-being is a very important aspect of recovery nursing. It is essential that nurses remember that individual patients need as much attention as the monitoring and other equipment that surrounds them.

Handover

Normally, patients who have had a general anaesthetic will still be unconscious when admitted to the recovery area following surgery. The anaesthetist should escort the patient to the recovery bay with the anaesthetic record and any drug or fluid charts. It is vital that nurses are in receipt of *all* relevant information about patients in their care and to this end, liaison between circulating and recovery nurses further improves continuity. In some day surgery units, nursing is organized in such a way that nurses provide total care for patients throughout their stay, undertaking the circulating role during their patient's procedure, assuming responsibility for first-stage recovery and subsequent post-operative care.

In most cases, handover from the anaesthetist will be to a designated recovery nurse and therefore must provide:

- details of the patient's name, type of anaesthetic used, the procedure performed and the name of the anaesthetist and surgeon
- details of the patient's condition including pre-existing disease and any potential airway or circulatory problems
- details of significant pre-operative factors – problems with deafness, hearing aids, anxiety levels
- postoperative instructions including oxygen therapy, monitoring, intravenous fluids and medications
- instructions for the management of postoperative pain.

Only when both the anaesthetist and recovery nurse are satisfied with the condition of the patient, then the anaesthetist may leave to continue their list. Relevant monitoring equipment, which is usually a pulse oximeter, should be connected immediately. The first priority for nursing assessment and management is the patient's airway and breathing. The assessment should include observation and documentation of:

- colour (lips, tongue, nail beds)
- pulse oximeter reading
- chest movement and pattern of breathing
- abnormal sounds, noisy breathing (snoring, stridor) – indicates partial obstruction
- movement of air with respiratory effort.

The essential nature of this observation cannot be overstated; simply looking at the pulse oximeter reading is not enough as the measurements are only accurate when the patient is well perfused (Hatfield & Tronson 1992). The method of airway management necessary largely depends on the type of anaesthetic each patient has received. In day surgery settings, nurses will commonly have to:

- manually maintain the patient's airway ± airway
- manage a laryngeal mask airway
- manage an endotracheal tube.

Manual Maintenance of Patient's Airway ± Airway

All patients should be given oxygen via a suitable face mask. The airway is maintained utilizing the *jaw thrust* manoeuvre, which is achieved by applying forward pressure on the angle of the jaw on both sides. This brings the tongue forward from the posterior wall of the pharynx and so relieves obstruction in unconscious patients. This can be supplemented by the use of an oral or nasal airway in anaesthetized patients. Oral airways need to be removed as patients regain consciousness and should be avoided in those individuals with caps, crowns or bridges of their front teeth to prevent damage to expensive dentalwork.

Laryngeal Mask Airway

The laryngeal mask airway has revolutionized airway management both during and following surgery and is likely be the most common technique seen in day surgery recovery areas. Therefore, we recommend that all staff view the excellent training video on the use of this technique that is available from the manufacturer. On arrival in recovery, patients should be given oxygen via the laryngeal mask. The technique used for this may well differ between units but a simple T-piece arrangement as shown previously (page 153) allows the patient to be supplied with a choice of oxygen concentrations. The mask is removed as the patient regains consciousness; patients tend to start to swallow before their protective reflexes return (Hatfield & Tronson 1992). This is a good sign to observe for it gives a good indication of when to remove the tube and ensures minimal distress to patients. When using the armoured variety of laryngeal mask it is worthwhile inserting an oral airway into the patient's mouth prior to their regaining consciousness. This prevents the patient biting and damaging the armoured component of the mask during their recovery.

Manage an Endotracheal Tube

This should be relatively uncommon scenario in a day unit recovery area. However, there should be the facility to look after a patient who, due to unforeseen circumstances, requires a short period of ventilation following their operation. However, this should only be for a short period and so the facility to transfer patients to an appropriate area for postoperative ventilation should be available.

Monitoring

During the time that patients are in the recovery area they must be kept under *continuous observation: the unconscious patient is unable to support their own airway.* We outlined in Chapter 6 the need for clear and uncluttered nursing documentation and first-stage recovery is a case in point. Care plans must be laid out in such a way to allow for easy recording of:

- time and frequency of recording observations
- oxygen saturation
- respiratory rate
- heart rate and rhythm
- blood pressure
- conscious level
- adequacy of pain relief
- drugs administered
- review of operation site.

The frequency of monitoring and recording the above is dependent on individual patient's condition and speed of recovery. Although protocols are useful for establishing baseline requirements, they are no substitute for close observation and sound clinical judgement. Hatfield and Tronson (1992) provide a useful outline of the patient's perception of their recovery which has clear implications for nursing practice:

- hearing returns first – voices of those around can seem particularly loud, distorted and often quite disturbing
- lights seem unduly bright, hurting the eyes and vision is blurred
- limbs feel heavy
- severe pain may be experienced
- memory returns but disorientation may continue.

Transient restlessness and agitation on emerging from anaesthesia is quite common (West 1992) but more common in children than adults (Drain 1994). Although restraint should not be used as a rule as it tends to increase patients' agitation (West 1992), children sometimes require *extremely gentle* restraint to protect them from injury. Make sure the sides of the trolley are raised at all times and are fitted with cushioned protectors. Gentle reassurance and orientation is essential and the restlessness usually subsides quite quickly. Parents should be encouraged to come into recovery if this will assist in settling their child.

Although quite common, it is still important to differentiate emergence restlessness from that associated with hypoxia, a full bladder or pain (Drain 1994); this is especially important with elderly patients with whom postoperative confusion is too often simply attributed to their age. Avoid sudden noises and do not shout. The elderly often take more time to recover, so allow more time; gentle and repeated orientation to time and place and early return of spectacles and dentures will help patients 'feel' more normal and facilitate communication.

Sometimes, patients will cry on waking from anaesthesia but it is not necessarily an indication that they are in pain. For instance, elderly people frequently have a greater tolerance for pain (Burden 1993). According to Hatfield and Tronson (1992) crying and unexplained distress can indicate that the patient was fully or partially aware during the surgical procedure. They also suggest that unpremedicated patients, those who are anxious and those anaesthetized with propofol are more likely to cry on wakening. These criteria clearly fit many day surgery patients so recovery staff should not be surprised by crying. Whatever the cause, all patients need support and appropriate reassurance. Speak quietly and evenly, calling the patient by their chosen name and use simple language to explain any monitoring you are doing. Be prepared to repeat the information as disorientation clearly interferes with information processing.

Discharge from Recovery

Criteria for discharge of patients from the recovery area should be established with the anaesthetic department. These should be based around those published by the Association of Anaesthetists (1993). Nursing staff must be satisfied that:

- the patient is conscious, can maintain a clear airway and protective reflexes are present
- breathing and oxygenation are satisfactory
- the cardiovascular system (pulse and blood pressure) is stable with no unexplained cardiac irregularity or persisting bleeding
- adequate analgesic and antiemetic provisions are made
- there is no evidence of hypothermia or hyperthermia.

Once these discharge criteria (plus any special requests by the anaesthetist) have been met then the patient may be discharged to the ward area of the unit. The responsibility for patient care is then passed on to the nurse who will continue to be responsible for their care until discharge. A formal handover should be completed similar to that used for the admission of the patient to the recovery area. *Always inform patients that you are about to move them.*

Management of Emergencies

In this section we consider the management of emergencies that may arise in the anaesthetic room, theatre or recovery area in which you may become involved. The emergencies covered will include:

- *Airway*
  obstruction – partial or complete
  respiratory arrest
  difficult intubation
  bronchospasm
  pneumothorax
- *Cardiovascular*
  hypotension
  dysrhythmias
  cardiac arrest
  anaphylaxis/anaphylactoid reactions

- *General*
  haemorrhage
  seizures
  malignant hyperpyrexia
  scoline apnoea.

Learning Points

Whilst the overall aim of this section is to provide clear guidelines for action in a variety of emergency situations, the importance of continued emotional support of patients in what can be quite terrifying situations cannot be overemphasized.

- Just as hearing is the last of the senses to be lost with the administration of a general anaesthetic, it is frequently the first to return.
- Think carefully about the impact of words and phrases and how they may be misinterpreted by waking patients.
- Use positive statements, reaffirming their recovery and your presence and support.
- Gentle yet purposive handling and care and communicating in a quiet and measured manner are essential to maintain patients' trust.

Airway Obstruction

It is vital that all nursing staff are able to recognize the signs of airway obstruction quickly and take immediate action to relieve it. It can be recognized by:

- observing patients' colour (lips, tongue, nail beds) – are they cyanosed?
- observing the pulse oximeter reading – is it low or falling?
- looking at patient's chest and observe the pattern of breathing – is the patient struggling to breathe? Is the chest expanding and the abdomen being sucked in? (this is known as rocking boat breathing and is evidence of obstruction)
- listening for abnormal sounds, noisy breathing (snoring, gurgling or stridor) – this indicates partial obstruction
- feeling for movement of air with respiratory effort.

Action

Give oxygen via a suitable face mask. Use the jaw thrust manoeuvre to bring the tongue away from the posterior wall of the pharynx. If this does not help and the patient is still unconscious, then insert an oral airway and again use the jaw thrust manoeuvre.

Stridor

Stridor in patients recovering from anaesthesia is usually caused by the presence of blood, sputum or secretions irritating the vocal cords.

Learning Point

- Oral airways should not be used in patients who are waking.
- They can stimulate the pharynx and cause laryngospasm or coughing. It is vital that you do not convey any more fear to the patient who is wakening and having difficulty breathing.
- A nasal airway should be used in this situation.

Action

If stridor is suspected, turn the patient into the left lateral position, tilted head down and suck out any blood or secretions using a soft suction catheter. If none of these techniques help the obstruction, then continue to attempt to optimize the airway *and* call for assistance from both anaesthetist and nursing colleagues to bring necessary airway management equipment and drugs (such as suxamethonium). If the anaesthetist is unable to maintain a clear airway or if the patient has obstructed completely (e.g. due to laryngospasm) suxamethonium may be given (to paralyse the patient) and the patient intubated with an endotracheal tube.

Respiratory Arrest

In the recovery area the most likely cause of respiratory arrest will be opioids given either during surgery or postoperatively in the recovery area; rapid assessment is vital. Respiratory arrest can be recognized quickly by following the observation process already discussed; that is:

- observing patients colour (lips, tongue, nail beds) – are they cyanosed?
- observing the pulse oximeter reading – is it low or falling?
- observing chest movements and pattern of breathing – is there evidence of respiratory movement?
- listening for sounds of breathing
- feeling for movement of air at the mouth and nose – is there any?

Action

Having established the diagnosis of respiratory arrest, assistance from both colleagues and anaesthetist should be summoned immediately. If the patient has a laryngeal mask airway, connect it to a breathing system or self-inflating bag and ventilate the patient using oxygen. If the patient does not have a laryngeal mask, insert an oral airway and ventilate the patient with oxygen using a breathing system or self-inflating bag and a facemask. The patient's oxygen saturation, pulse and blood pressure should be monitored throughout and an ECG connected if there is any dysrhythmia. The effectiveness of the ventilation can be quickly assessed from the pulse oximeter reading. Nursing colleagues should bring the airway equipment and a supply of naloxone and doxapram which may be requested by the anaesthetist. The anaesthetist will take over management of the airway and assess why the patient has had a respiratory arrest. Appropriate treatment may then be started.

Difficult Intubation

Although possible, this situation is unlikely to be met in the recovery room of a day unit. However, it may occur in the anaesthetic room and the assistance of the recovery staff may be requested. In day surgery, difficult intubation should not be an emergency situation as the patient is fasted and is scheduled for elective surgery. Having established that the patient is difficult (or impossible!) to intubate the anaesthetist has a number of choices, for example:

- wake the patient and provide a local anaesthetic technique for the operation
- insert a laryngeal mask and proceed with the operation
- request further equipment to achieve the intubation.

It is this latter course that may lead to the involvement of the recovery staff and it is important that you are aware of where the secondary airway management equipment is stored in your area.

Bronchospasm

Bronchospasm may be seen on its own or as part of an anaphylactoid reaction; therefore, it is important to look for the presence of other signs of anaphylactoid reactions mentioned later in this chapter. Bronchospasm is the term used to describe the wheeze experienced by patients who have asthma, though it may occur in non-asthmatic patients.

Action

If a patient sounds wheezy whilst still unconscious you should:

- give the patient oxygen
- check the patient's observations – pulse, blood pressure and oxygen saturation
- assess the amount of difficulty the patient is having with breathing
- ensure the upper airway is not obstructed
- listen to the patient's chest with a stethoscope – listen for a wheeze on expiration and a prolonged expiratory time.

If listening to the chest confirms the signs of bronchospasm or if you are unhappy with the level of wheeze then inform the anaesthetist immediately. Severe bronchospasm results in very little air entry to the lungs despite massive respiratory effort, in the absence of any upper airway obstruction; it clearly requires more urgent management. You should request help from the anaesthetist immediately and ask for appropriate nebulizing equipment and salbutamol to be prepared and brought to the bay. The anaesthetist should assess the patient, start suitable treatment and remain with the patient until you are happy to take responsibility for the patient once more. The patient must not leave recovery until the bronchospasm has settled.

Pneumothorax

Pneumothorax is not a likely complication to be found in day surgery. This, however, makes it even more difficult to recognize as to diagnose the problem one first must be aware of the possibility! Signs to look for include:

- uneven expansion of the chest
- increasing respiratory effort
- dyspnoea
- fall in oxygen saturation
- fall in blood pressure
- patient complaining of pain in the chest.

The diagnosis can be confirmed by listening to the chest – absence of breath sounds on the affected side will be noted. It is worth noting that there are two types of pneumothorax that the patient may have – simple or tension. The tension pneumothorax is more dangerous and life-threatening as pressure builds up in the affected side pushing the mediastinum (and so the heart) across against the other lung. This causes major disturbances to the patient's oxygenation and blood pressure and the tension must be released urgently.

Action

Request assistance from the anaesthetist immediately. The anaesthetist will confirm the diagnosis and manage the problem appropriately – in the case of a tension pneumothorax a canula will be inserted into the affected side to relieve the pressure and so improve the condition of the patient. Then a chest drain can be inserted in a controlled, less urgent fashion.

Hypotension

The discovery of hypotension following anaesthesia is not unusual and this is one of the more common situations you will encounter. The golden rule in assessing hypotension is '*never trust a single blood pressure reading*'. Always recheck the blood pressure and check the patient's care plan to establish the pre-operative recording.

Action

If this confirms that the patient *is* hypotensive then note pulse (rate and rhythm) and oxygen saturation, give oxygen via a suitable face mask and check the patient's operation site for haemorrhage. Management should then be guided by the degree of hypotension present. Mild hypotension (i.e. a systolic pressure within 25% of the patient's normal or above 80 mmHg) – pass the observations listed above to the anaesthetist with a request for advice. If the hypotension is more severe than this then:

- ensure patient is receiving oxygen
- call the anaesthetist to review the patient
- speed up the administration of intravenous fluids (if present)
- consider elevating the patient's legs to aid venous return.

The anaesthetist should then review the patient as a matter of urgency and decide on appropriate further management.

Dysrhythmias

Before considering further the management of dysrhythmias, it is important to define what is meant by dysrhythmia (or arrhythmia). 'Dys' has a Greek derivation and means 'bad' or 'ill' which may be a more appropriate description than the 'a' prefix which is Greek for 'no' or 'not' (i.e. in medicine this prefix is used to denote the absence of something! The patient's pulse perhaps?) In this section we consider rhythm disturbances such as:

- tachycardia greater than 110
- bradycardia less than 50
- irregular pulse.

If you observe any pulse irregularities you must consider whether this is a *new* phenomenon; that is, has this patient had this problem since admission? A quick review of the patient's care plan should provide this information, and if the patient is taking any cardiac drugs. Those drugs potentially linked to a history of dysrhythmias include verapamil, digoxin and β-blockers.

Action

Give the patient oxygen and check blood pressure and oxygen saturation. If the patient is awake ask them if they have any symptoms of chest pain or breathlessness, but be careful not to frighten them by asking these questions. Further management will clearly depend on the answers.

- *If the patient was admitted with a dysrhythmia.* If the patient's condition is stable, blood pressure and saturation are normal and the patient has no symptoms, then continue with management as normal.
- *If the patient was not admitted with a dysrhythmia.* Again, if the patient's condition is stable, blood pressure and saturation are normal and they have no symptoms, continue with management as normal *but inform the anaesthetist about this new finding.* If the patient is not stable, is hypotensive or complaining of chest pain or breathlessness, then ask the anaesthetist to review the patient urgently and begin ECG monitoring.

Cardiac Arrest

Cardiac arrest is a situation where the patient is in asystole or ventricular fibrillation. The diagnosis of cardiac arrest can be difficult and it is important to make the diagnosis quickly so that basic and advanced life-support measures can be promptly instituted. The signs include:

- loss of a palpable carotid pulse
- loss of consciousness in the patient who has been awake
- loss of pulse oximeter reading
- inability of blood pressure monitor to measure patient's blood pressure
- characteristic ECG monitor trace (if monitored) flat line of asystole, chaotic activity of ventricular fibrillation.

Action

Having made the diagnosis you must:

- send for medical help – sound the emergency call system
- recruit help from all available colleagues in recovery
- ventilate the patient with 100% oxygen via bag and mask, or laryngeal mask if this is already *in situ*
- ensure colleagues have brought the arrest equipment including the defibrillator to the patient
- organize a colleague to start cardiac massage.

At this stage medical help should have arrived. Resuscitation should follow Resuscitation Council (UK) guidelines (Basic Life Support Working Party of the European Resuscitation Council 1992; Advanced Life Support Working Party of the European Resuscitation Council 1992) and the recovery area should have a copy of the resuscitation nomogram easily visible.

Anaphylaxis/Anaphylactoid Reactions

Anaphylaxis occurs when a patient has developed an immune response (sensitivity) to a substance (a drug or even a foodstuff such as peanuts) which is known as the antigen. Having been exposed to this antigen once the patient develops an antibody (IgE) to it. When exposed to the substance again, the antibody reacts with it and causes a severe reaction known as anaphylaxis. The antibody and antigen react together causing a massive release of histamine and other mediators from mast cells in the body. These provoke the classic signs and symptoms of anaphylaxis. These are:

- pruritis
- urticaria
- dyspnoea
- bronchospasm
- nausea and vomiting
- hypotension
- cyanosis
- airway problems may occur.

Action

Treatment needs to be instituted quickly, particularly if the reaction occurs to some intravenous drugs such as sodium thiopentone. Treatment includes:

- administration of oxygen
- administration of adrenaline
- maintain or establish secure airway
- establish intravenous access if not already present
- administration of intravenous fluids, further adrenaline as necessary and steroids.

A useful treatment chart that is laminated and suitable for hanging on anaesthetic machines and in recovery bays is produced by the Association of Anaesthetists.

Haemorrhage

Haemorrhage can occur in two forms: it may be concealed or revealed. Concealed haemorrhage occurs when the patient is bleeding into an area that is not visible, for example into their abdomen following a laparoscopy. Therefore, in this situation the first sign you will notice is tachycardia and then hypotension. However, it is important to realize that in fit young patients these signs, and hypotension in particular, do not occur until the patient has lost a considerable amount of blood. A young fit patient of average weight may have lost more than 800 ml of blood before developing a tachycardia and 1500 ml before their blood pressure falls. Therefore, it can be difficult to diagnose concealed haemorrhage. In the event of unexplained tachycardia and/or hypotension you must consider blood loss. Think of the procedure the patient has undergone – could it lead to concealed blood loss?

Action

Early notification and discussion of the patient with both the anaesthetist and surgeon should be considered. The patient with marked hypotension should be managed within the guidelines for revealed haemorrhage.

Revealed haemorrhage is much easier to diagnose! In this situation the patient will be bleeding from the operative site. This allows measurement of the blood loss in most, but not all, situations. Bleeding following tonsillectomy, though revealed, is notoriously difficult to quantify. Haemorrhage following surgery sufficient to soak through the dressings over the operation site is not uncommon following some procedures. However, continued blood loss and the requirement to dress the wound repeatedly is not normal in the recovery area. In this situation, the patient should remain in the recovery area until the staff are satisfied that the problem has settled. Early discussion with the surgeon is advised.

Action

In the event of sudden large blood loss resulting in hypotension you should:

- call for assistance from the anaesthetist
- give the patient oxygen and ensure their airway and breathing are satisfactory
- apply pressure to the affected area – control the haemorrhage if possible
- speed up the intravenous fluids if present or if not, then run through an intravenous line for the anaesthetist (use 1 l of Hartmann's solution)
- ensure that the patient's blood pressure, oxygen saturation and ECG are monitored and recorded
- if the patient's blood pressure falls below 80 mmHg then consider elevating the patient's legs.

Learning Point

- The use of head-down tilt though offering the benefit of increasing venous return to the heart may theoretically reduce cerebral blood flow due to the back pressure from the venous circulation.

Seizures

Seizures do occur in the recovery period and knowledge of their management is important for recovery staff. However, they may well be an unusual occurrence in day surgery as many units refuse to treat susceptible patients as day cases. At pre-admission assessment this can be achieved by only allowing stable epileptic patients who have had previous anaesthesia with no problems to be cared for as day cases. Epileptic patients should be told to continue taking their medication as normal including on the day of surgery.

Action

In the event of a seizure occurring you should:

- send for assistance – colleagues nearby and the anaesthetist
- ensure the patient is not harming themselves on the sides of the trolley
- position the patient on their left side with head-down tilt if possible
- protect the patient's airway
- give oxygen
- organize a colleague to draw up a syringe of 20 mg of diazepam.

Malignant Hyperpyrexia

Malignant hyperpyrexia is a rare disease (1 in 50 000) that has a genetic basis and so may occur in the blood relatives of a sufferer. The incidence in children is 1 in 14 000, making it three times greater than in adults (Burden 1993). The patient who is susceptible to this problem often does not realize this as susceptibility may skip a generation (the disease is characterized by dominant inheritance with incomplete penetrance). Furthermore, it does not effect their normal lives and it is only when exposed to 'trigger' agents that they are put in danger. The most important trigger agents are the volatile anaesthetic agents and suxamethonium – though there are others. Early diagnosis and treatment is vital in the management of this condition which carries a high mortality rate. Staff must therefore be aware of the condition and know what to do.

Clinical features include:

- raised temperature ($>2°C$ per hour)
- muscle rigidity
- tachycardia
- tachypnoea
- reduced oxygen saturation with cyanosis
- raised end tidal CO_2.

Action

In the event of suspicion of a recovery patient having this problem you must:

- check the patient's temperature
- check their heart rate in recovery and theatre – has it increased?
- check their oxygen saturation – is it falling?
- check their respiratory rate – is it rapid?

Once the results of these are obtained the staff should discuss the patient quickly with the anaesthetist. Management of malignant hyperpyrexia includes:

- curtailing surgery and anaesthesia – if diagnosis made in theatre
- give the patient 100% oxygen – helps counteract the massive O_2 consumption
- establish intravenous infusion – use cooled fluids if possible and avoid Hartmann's
- monitor the patient's temperature, pulse, saturation, ECG and blood pressure
- institute surface cooling – use ice packs in axillae and groin
- check blood gases and electrolytes – patient may require ventilation
- give bicarbonate and dextrose/insulin as indicated to control acidosis and hyperkalaemia
- give intravenous *dantrolene* – the usual dose is 4 mg kg^{-1}
- promote diuresis – renal and cardiac failure are constant threats (Hatfield & Tronson 1992).

The management of this condition requires the recovery staff and at least one anaesthetist to work together as a team. The operating session should be cancelled or discontinued until the patient is stabilized and transferred to intensive care. Recovery staff do not need to know the complex management of this rare condition by heart but excellent guidelines for its management are available as posters from the manufacturers of dantrolene. It is vital that recovery staff know what to do in the event of this rare condition and know where the supply of dantrolene is kept in their hospital; clearly, this essential but expensive drug must be kept in an accessible place.

Suxamethonium (Scoline) Apnoea

Suxamethonium is a drug used by anaesthetists to paralyse patients for a short period. It causes the patient considerable muscle aches and pains in the days following its use, particularly in young, fit ambulant patients. Therefore, its use in day surgery should be kept to a minimum and this condition should rarely be seen in day surgery. However, there is some evidence that one of the newer muscle relaxants mivacurium, which may well be used in day surgery, may cause a similar problem in the same group of susceptible patients.

Susceptible patients have a problem with the enzyme (serum cholinesterase) that metabolizes these drugs. Serum cholinesterase serves no real purpose in the body and so its absence or the presence of an abnormal variant of it does not cause the patient any problems. Exposure to these drugs, however, leads to a paralysis that can last for many hours. The condition should be recognized in theatre by the anaesthetist at the end of the operation, as typically patients fail to start breathing for themselves. The anaesthetist will then use a peripheral nerve stimulator to assess the degree of nerve block present. If this supports the diagnosis then the patient requires ventilation (probably on an intensive care unit) and should be kept asleep until the paralysis wears off.

There are several different types of variant of cholinesterase and the time taken for the problem to resolve can vary from one to several hours. Providing it is spotted and the patient remains ventilated and asleep, then the condition is not life threatening. Patients should have blood tests performed to confirm the diagnosis and assess the genetic type of the variant they have. Following confirmation of the condition, patients' blood relatives need to have the blood tests performed and to be advised of the result.

Summary

There is a strong argument for ensuring that all nurses working in a day surgery unit are able to work safely in the recovery area. However, it is also important to recognize that the first-stage recovery is a *critical care* area and requires a core complement of fully trained staff who are prepared to teach and assess the necessary skills to their peers. However, all nurses must recognize the potentially deleterious effects of unrelieved anxiety and the importance of providing psychological and emotional support to patients during this period. Although many of the emergencies discussed here are thankfully rare occurrences in day surgery (as a result of rigorous selection processes and anaesthetic criteria), it remains essential that staff working in this area ensure that their knowledge of normal and abnormal physiology and pharmacology is appropriate to the patients they are caring for.

Key Points

- First-stage recovery areas are classified as critical care areas and should be staffed appropriately.
- Trusts are responsible for ensuring that recommendations for monitoring and other equipment needs for each patient are met.
- Nurses are responsible for checking all drugs and necessary equipment prior to each list.
- The anaesthetist caring for a patient continues to be responsible for that patient until they have recovered sufficiently to be returned to the ward.
- Anaesthetized patients must be supervised at all times: the unconscious patient is unable to support their own airway.
- Psychological and emotional support of patients is just as important as the more technical aspects of management.
- Close observation and immediate, accurate interpretation of abnormal signs is essential in managing emergencies.

Recommended Reading

Hatfield, A. and Tronson, M. (1992) **The Complete Recovery Room Book.** Oxford: OUP

An excellent text. The book is well laid out, highlights vital areas appropriately and covers all aspects of recovery care

NATN (1995) **Operating Department Practitioners, NVQ Level 3: the new updated standards. A statement from NATN.** *British Journal of Theatre Nursing* **5**(7): 10–11.

Havill, C. and Walker, J. (1994) **Working together – National Vocational Qualification in operating department practice.** *Surgical Nurse* **7**(4): 9–13

These two articles provide further information regarding the preparation of operating department personnel, the standards required of programmes and some of the benefits of shared education and collaborative working

References

Advanced Life Support Working Party of the European Resuscitation Council (1992) **Guidelines for Advanced Life Support.** *Resuscitation* **24**: 111–121.

Association of Anaesthetists (1985) **Working party on postanaesthetic recovery facilities.** Association of Anaesthetists.

Association of Anaesthetists (1993) **Immediate postanaesthetic recovery.** Association of Anaesthetists.

Basic Life Support Working Party of the European Resuscitation Council (1992) **Guidelines for basic life support.** *Resuscitation* **24**: 103–110.

Burden, N. (1993) **Ambulatory Surgical Nursing.** Philadelphia: WB Saunders.

DHSS (1983) **Ventilation of operating departments – A design guide.** DHSS Engineering Data DV/4.

Drain, C. B. (1992) **The Post Anaesthesia Care Unit: A critical care unit approach to post anaesthesia nursing** (Third Edition). Philadelphia: WB Saunders.

Drain, C. B. (1994) **The Post Anaesthesia Care Unit: A critical care approach to post anaesthesia nursing** (Third Edition). Philadelphia: WB Saunders.

Farman, J. V. (1978) **The work of the recovery room.** *British Journal of Hospital Medicine* **19**: 606–616.

Hatfield, A. and Tronson, M. (1992) **The Complete Recovery Room Book.** Oxford: OUP.

Hudson, R. B. S. (1979) **Pattern of work in the recovery room.** *Journal of the Royal Society of Medicine* **4**: 273–275.

Utting, J. E. in Johnston, I. D. A. and Hunter, A. R. (Eds) (1984) **The Design and Utilisation of Operating Theatres.** London: Edward Arnold

Ward, C. S. (1985) **Anaesthetic Equipment.** London: Baillière Tindall.

West, B. J. M. (1992) **Theatre Nursing. Technique and Care** (Sixth Edition). London: Baillière Tindall.

Chapter 11 Postoperative management, discharge and follow-up care

Overview

This chapter is concerned with the ongoing postoperative management and care of patients following completion of their surgical procedure, and emphasizes the importance of continued observation and monitoring. Care during this postoperative period is generally the responsibility of ward-based nurses and the variety of different settings in which it may take place are explored, as are their advantages and disadvantages. However, regardless of how a day surgery unit might manage ongoing care, problem-free recovery and successful discharge is dependent on skilled nursing care and meticulous organization. A proactive approach to postoperative pain and nausea and vomiting is essential for a successful patient outcome and some strategies for managing these more common complications associated with day surgery are evaluated. This chapter continues to advocate continuity of care and early involvement of patients' carers in relation to discharge preparation and management and offers suggestions for post-discharge support and follow-up.

Chapter Focus

- Organization of postoperative management
- Postoperative needs of patients
- Managing pain and nausea and vomiting
- Return to normality and criteria for discharge
- Problems associated with discharge
- Ongoing support and follow-up

Introduction

Qualified nurses undertaking post-registration education in day surgery (ENB A21) frequently and consistently identify the postoperative period as the time when the 'conveyor belt' experience can be felt acutely by patients. It is essential that patients are able to recover safely in their own time, but too often, they can feel that they are under some pressure to get up and go home, even when no explicit words to that effect have been spoken. Therefore, the environment in which ongoing care takes place, the organization of postoperative management and nurses' activities during this period are worth considering in order that possible reasons for patients' perceptions can be identified and the quality of care maximized.

Organizing Postoperative Management

Day surgery units frequently differ in their design and layout, organization of patient care facilities, and delivery of care. For example, some units will opt for beds for patients to recover on, others will have trolleys or reclining chairs, and some a mixture of all three. All options have their strengths and weaknesses; patient comfort, capital investment and moving and handling implications are necessary considerations in decision-making and selection. There is little doubt that for most surgical procedures, beds promote rest and provide the most comfortable option for patients. However, hospital beds reinforce the 'patient role' and as Burden (1993) points out, they do not encourage patients to move nor do they promote 'normality'. Similarly, day units need to adopt a model of ongoing care that matches not only the individual geographical layout of a unit, availability of nursing skills, range and number of procedures undertaken and individual anaesthetic and surgical protocols, but also the philosophy of day surgery. For example, if patients continue to be prescribed premedication, they must be transferred to theatre on a trolley; this follows the inpatient model. As we have seen, most patients do not require premedication for day surgery procedures and are therefore able to walk to theatre, thereby promoting greater independence and feelings of normality.

There is no definitive method of organizing postoperative care in a day surgery setting. Providing essential safety requirements are met, there are many possible individual variations, but two major organizational models appear to predominate:

The ward setting – pre- and postoperative care carried out in a typical 'ward' environment, fitted out with either beds or trolleys. Patients spend the necessary minimum time in first-stage recovery before returning to the ward area for ongoing observation and care. This most closely resembles the traditional inpatient model, and some of the advantages and disadvantages of the arrangement are outlined in Box 11.1.

The lounge setting – pre- and postoperative care takes place in 'lounge' areas furnished with easy/reclining chairs. Patients spend a greater length of time in first-stage recovery and return to continue to recover in a easy chair. This approach resembles the 'Phase II' care commonly adopted in ambulatory surgery units in the USA (Burden 1993). The advantages and disadvantages of such 'lounge style' areas are outlined in Box 11.2.

Box 11.1 Advantages and disadvantages of 'ward style' postoperative areas

Advantages

- Provides a 'familiar' environment, often utilizing an existing ward area and therefore assuring that necessary oxygen and suction apparatus is available
- First-stage recovery area can deal with a greater number of patients as throughput is faster
- Recovery nursing staff are providing first-stage recovery care in line with training and experience

Disadvantages

- As nurses take up familiar position behind some kind of 'desk' or station, it does not promote nurse–patient interaction
- Lying on beds in straight lines reinforces the patient role and hospital environment and does not encourage interaction between patients
- Unless a third-stage area is available, early involvement of relatives/carers is not possible

Box 11.2 Advantages and disadvantages of 'lounge style' postoperative areas

Advantages

- Reinforces the philosophy of day surgery as a different and more patient-orientated approach to care
- Promotes interaction between patients and early involvement of relatives
- Lounge areas can be less 'technical' in appearance and therefore less threatening environments for many patients – with thought and planning, essential oxygen/suction apparatus and call systems can be installed in less obvious ways
- Use of recliner chairs encourages both patient activity and return to normality – a more normal position in which to drink a cup of tea and enjoy some hot toast!

Disadvantages

- Can promote the inaccurate assumption that patients in chairs somehow require less observation and support
- More time in first-stage recovery reduces the number of patients on a list
- Therefore there is the tendency by some units to staff these postoperative areas with untrained staff
- Difficulty in ensuring privacy for patients in the event of delayed effects of anaesthesia or surgery
- If relatives are invited in, the noise level for other patients can be uncomfortable
- Inappropriate use/volume of television and radio
- Can become crowded if area serves multipurpose uses

It could be argued that the physical surroundings, furniture and model of organization are less important in creating a safe supportive environment for patients than the skills and commitment of individual nurses. However, the ideal would combine the two with provision of ward-based care and a postoperative lounge area in which patients can be prepared for discharge in the company of their relatives. All such areas require supervision by trained nurses who can recognize the onset of untoward symptoms and initiate appropriate action.

Regardless of individual differences, *all* second-stage postoperative areas must ensure the following are provided:

- sufficient staffing to facilitate ongoing observation
- adequate oxygen and suction points
- means of monitoring blood pressure
- even, diffused light
- quiet atmosphere
- privacy
- warmth
- adequate fresh air
- ample bathroom and toilet facilities
- nurse call/emergency system.

Learning Point

- All postoperative areas require supervision by trained nurses who can recognize the onset of untoward symptoms and initiate appropriate action.

With the use of contemporary anaesthetic agents such as *propofol* increasing, recovery from general anaesthesia is generally quite rapid and free of previously common symptoms such as headache and drowsiness. However, as pointed out in Chapter 8, patients' responses to anaesthesia can be unpredictable and it is important to adhere to accepted protocols.

Principles of Postoperative Management in Day Surgery

We suggest that the general postoperative needs of day surgery patients are essentially no different than those of inpatients, except of course that our patient group is required to get up and go home within a much shorter time. Therefore, ensuring that postoperative recovery is complete and free of complications is a clear priority. We make no apology for emphasizing postoperative needs in this way as it helps to reinforce two important points:

- that day surgery patients require the same attention as any other patients in terms of their physical and psychological comfort
- these are elements of care that can really underline the quality of the service provided.

It might be useful here to return to Orem's model (1991) to review the specific postoperative requirements of day surgery patients. In Chapter 6, we identified Orem's six universal care needs as:

- sufficient intake of water, air and food
- prevention of hazards
- balance between activity and rest
- maintenance of elimination
- balance between social interaction and rest
- promotion of development and potential.

Intake of Air, Water and Food

Air

Ongoing observation of the patient's condition on return from first-stage recovery is essential. Although complications at this stage are quite rare, it is still important that patients continue to *feel* supported during this time and for nurses to ensure that cardiovascular and respiratory status remains normal. This requires frequent observation and monitoring and nurses should be with the patients, not observing from a distance. Observation from a static sitting position (normally behind a desk of some sort) is of little value, even less so when trolley sides are up and the patients are laid on their side. Some units insist that one nurse must always be in the room with patients in the postoperative phase, which is not really necessary – it is not common practice on inpatient surgical wards and if patients require that amount of supervision they should still be in first-stage recovery. We do, however, argue strongly for ongoing observation to ensure that patients are still breathing, are well perfused and recovering normally.

Water

A small number of patients, depending upon their surgical procedure, will require intravenous fluids in the immediate postoperative period. Most patients, however, have undergone procedures that incur little or no fluid loss and are therefore able to start taking oral fluids as soon as they are sufficiently awake and feel like doing so. Despite many patients' protestations to the contrary, it makes sense to start with a small amount of water and, if tolerated well, then offer a cup of tea. Milk, coffee and fruit juices (especially cordials) are associated with inducing nausea and should be avoided where possible. Personal experience suggests more use of herbal teas; peppermint or camomile are good options but only if already enjoyed under more normal circumstances and they are unlikely to prove popular with children. Parents and the children themselves are usually the best arbiters of what is an appropriate postoperative drink, but very sweet drinks are probably best avoided. Specific nursing management and treatment of postoperative nausea and vomiting is to be found later in this chapter.

Food

In Chapters 7 and 8 we highlighted that excessive fasting is frequently associated with nausea postoperatively, especially in children. Early introduction of solid food is beneficial both physiologically (can help reduce nausea) and psychologically (promotes and reinforces the sense of returning normality). We have found that toast is universally popular amongst patients of all ages and the smell of its preparation usually acts as an appetite stimulant rather than the opposite. Depending on the time of day, soup and sandwiches are good options, but fillings should be quite light and bland.

Elimination

Royle and Walsh (1992) suggest that under normal circumstances adequately hydrated surgical patients will pass urine within 6–8 h of surgery. Most day surgery patients fit into this category and have no problem passing urine spontaneously and, depending on the procedure carried out, usually prior to going home. Thankfully, day surgery nurses do not appear to exhibit the almost obsessional preoccupation with patients' bladder-emptying activities that is often to be found on inpatient wards. However, it is still worth identifying briefly the factors that affect patients' ability to pass urine postoperatively; these are outlined in Box 11.3.

In most instances, once patients have had time to rest, have a drink and started to move around, the desire to pass urine will return. Therefore, bed pans and urinals will usually not be necessary and in a room potentially full of other patients, neither are they appropriate. However, women having undergone D & C or other pelvic examinations sometimes have crampy period-like pains

Box 11.3 Factors contributing to temporary inability to pass urine

- Inhibitory effects of anaesthetic agents
- ? Small increase in anti-diuretic hormone (ADH) release as result of surgery and pre-operative anxiety
- Patient age and gender
- Individual patient history
- Type of surgical procedure performed
- Period of preoperative fasting
- Level of hydration
- Incidence and extent of any vomiting
- Postoperative position

after the procedure which can be accompanied by the need to pass urine. Similarly, older men who have had urological procedures feel the need to pass urine some time before they are able to get up to the toilet. The issue of what Burden (1993) refers to as 'urinary status' will be addressed once more in relation to discharge criteria later in this chapter.

Prevention of Hazards

In this section, the specific hazards we are looking at are shock and haemorrhage, pain, nausea and vomiting. Although other quite distressing symptoms can be felt such as dizziness, drowsiness or headache, they rarely delay or prevent discharge and usually settle with time, rest and compassionate nursing care.

Shock and Haemorrhage

Complications such as these are thankfully quite rare in most day surgery units. However, continuing to classify procedures as *minor* often implies minimal care required, but complacency with regard to patients' recovery is not something any of us can afford. So, whilst a one-off pulse recording may be all that many patients require, this will not always be the case. As more elderly and potentially less fit patients become acceptable for day surgery, postoperative observation must meet more stringent guidelines. But clearly, any patient who has remained in first-stage recovery for longer than normal, perhaps as a result of bleeding and/or hypotension, requires *ongoing* monitoring. Similarly, any patient who after sitting up looks pale and suddenly complains of feeling faint and nauseated needs urgent attention. Experience tells us that it is often other patients in the immediate vicinity who draw attention to those who have become unwell, underlining once more the importance of observation. In these instances:

- lie the patient down again gently
- observe surgical site for local signs of haemorrhage (in vaginal procedures – check sanitary pads carefully)
- monitor and record pulse and blood pressure at least twice in the first hour
- if hypotension persists and you suspect or confirm bleeding, inform the anaesthetist and the surgeon immediately
- act calmly and quietly to allay fear in both this patient and others nearby.

Meeting nurses from different day surgery units has provided us with the opportunity to assess the extent of variation in postoperative observations. Views appear quite polarized with one school of thought suggesting that no routine observations are necessary and the opposing view

Learning Points

- Although complications such as shock and haemorrhage are quite rare, complacency cannot be afforded.
- Ongoing monitoring of patients postoperatively is essential.
- Decisions to monitor vital signs should be based on assessment of the effects of anaesthesia on individual patients, *not* driven by procedure or tradition.

appearing to believe that anything less than half-hourly temperature, pulse, respirations (TPR) and blood pressure recordings for 4 h places patients lives in jeopardy. The 'correct' approach will always be the one in which decisions to monitor vital signs are based on knowledge and assessment of the effects of anaesthesia on individual patients rather than procedure-driven assessment and tradition.

Postoperative Pain

There is little doubt that postoperative pain following day surgery continues to be a common problem (Leith *et al.* 1994, Raistrick 1994, Ratcliffe *et al.* 1994, Wilkinson *et al.* 1992). Pain following surgery varies enormously. The nature of the surgical procedure appears to be the most significant determinant of both pain experience and requirements of analgesia, with laparascopic sterilization and some orthopaedic procedures high on the list of greater pain experiences of patients. As suggested in Chapter 8, our knowledge and understanding of pain and pain perception is increasing all the time and the adoption of more consistent approaches to pain management is undoubtedly having a significant impact on patient satisfaction with this element of day surgery. However, there are still too many clinicians and nurses who believe that certain procedures such as insertion of grommets and D & C are not painful. In the case of beliefs about the latter, these are individuals who have clearly never suffered the misery of severe dysmenorrhoea.

A non-judgemental, accepting approach and patient-centred assessment provides the key to effective pain control.

Only the person with pain can assess its severity. Any attempts by nurses to modify that assessment or put it into other words is devaluing that assessment. Sadly, too often we hear comments like '... well, she's rolling around the bed and saying that the pains terrible! But she's only had a D & C – she can't be in that much pain!'. Unfortunately, this error is compounded by

Box 11.4 Guidelines for managing patients' pain

Pre-operatively

- Discuss pain with patients to assess the impact of any previous experiences and strategies utilized
- Explain a simple visual pain score tool
- Encourage patient to report pain symptoms as soon as they occur
- Reassure that any pain they have will be managed promptly

Postoperatively

- Observe closely for non-verbal indicators of pain as patient recovers – e.g. restlessness, facial expression, crying, posture and position on trolley – especially important with young children
- Monitor effects on pulse and/or B/P
- Assist patient into more comfortable position with extra support from pillows as necessary – with a child, on to mum's lap for a cuddle is probably the best option
- Consider gentle massage or application of heat pad for backache or shoulder pain resulting from operative position
- Encourage patient to assess pain against pain score and to put pain into words on waking
- Dependent on assessment, give prescribed analgesia and monitor its effects
- Reassess with same pain score 30 min later

Learning Points

- Pain is an individual and unique experience.
- Individual patient assessment is essential.
- Nurses' and clinicians' own beliefs about what constitutes a painful procedure can seriously compromise patient care.
- A non-judgemental, accepting approach and patient-centred assessment provides the key to effective pain control.

the fact that is difficult for nurses who do not believe or accept patients' assessment of pain to keep it out of their faces and gestures, which will not go unnoticed by patients. This has implications for the quality of nurse–patient relationships and level of satisfaction with care.

As with most nurse–patient interactions, the general approach and communication skills adopted by nurses are just as important (if not more) as the specific intervention; that is, the *acceptance* of the pain, the *empathy* and the *time* are just as important as the analgesia.

Postoperative Nausea and Vomiting

Whilst poorly controlled pain is not surprisingly a major factor in determining the quality of patient outcome, there is little doubt that postoperative nausea and vomiting (PONV) can similarly delay or cancel discharge (Robinson D 1993). It is estimated that more than a third of all patients undergoing surgical procedures in the UK suffer from PONV (Medicare Audit 1993) and nurses could perhaps do more to improve the experience of patients with respect to this distressing and undignified symptom. For example, although Nightingale (1994) believes that the majority of nurses understand the distressing nature of PONV to patients, only one in three prescriptions for anti-emetics are ever given. Nurses, she argues, tend to adopt a 'wait and see' approach to the management of PONV rather than treat it prophylactically. The potential impact of PONV is not always appreciated by clinicians either, though more appears to be done in day surgery than in inpatient areas, largely as a result of the financial implications of admission.

As with pain, management of PONV begins pre-operatively. There are a number of different factors at play in the incidence of nausea and vomiting following surgery; some are within the patient, others are directly related to the surgery. Having greater understanding of such factors may help nurses identify those most at risk and plan their care appropriately. Ogg and Hitchcock (1994) identify the following surgical/anaesthetic factors:

- nature and length of surgical procedure – incidence in laparoscopy, knee arthroscopy and dental procedures is high
- pre-operative medication – not common practice for many procedures
- anaesthetic induction agent – lowered incidence with propofol
- anaesthetic maintenance agent
- muscle relaxant reversal – few are used for intermediate procedures
- postoperative analgesia – opiates increase incidence
- patient movement – rapid movement, e.g. sitting up too quickly, increases PONV.

Women are up to three times more likely to develop PONV than men, with children having double the incidence of adults (Robinson D 1993). Patients who have experienced PONV previously are more likely to suffer it again; those who are fasted excessively, those who are very anxious pre-operatively and those with a history of travel sickness or migraine are also at greater risk (Burden 1993).

Many of these factors can be identified and discussed at pre-admission assessment or immediately pre-operatively, but Burden (1993) warns that too much discussion of these factors may increase the chance of patients feeling nauseated. She argues that PONV is very much a self-fulfilling prophecy in that those patients who are convinced they will be sick usually will be, whereas those who can convince themselves that they will not (with the help of the nursing and medical staff) often are not. That said, these causal factors highlight some important principles of care:

- Prevention is better than treatment.
- Limit fasting times to minimum (see Chapter 7).
- Take note of predisposing factors in individual patients.
- Note type of surgery and use to predict PONV.
- Avoid sudden and rapid movement, e.g. elevating head quickly.
- Introduce fluids slowly, taking cue from how the patients feel. Do not decide that patients are ready to eat without asking them first (see Robinson, H. 1994).
- Give prescribed anti-emetic prophylactically whenever possible; do not wait for patients to vomit first.
- Do not leave a stack of vomit bowls for patients who are being sick – far from providing reassurance it gives two distinct messages: (1) they are going to be *very* sick (all those bowls to fill), and (2) you are not going to be back for a while.
- Take heed of patients need for privacy – no one wants to be sick in public.

Activity, Social Interaction and Rest

Back at the beginning of this chapter, we mentioned the conveyor belt experience and suggested that in order for patients to feel like they are on a production line, no words to that effect need to be spoken. The saying 'actions speak louder than words' is very relevant in this context and highlights the importance of matching non-verbal behaviour to verbal communication.

Patients can feel pressurized to get up and go home as a result of heightened activity in the ward area, references by nurses to lunch breaks, afternoon lists or things they still need to do, other patients getting up, etc. What we should be striving for is the creation of a climate in which patients are comfortable, understand their surgery and ongoing care, and their role and

Reflection Point

Consider the following scenario . . .

11.50 hrs

Nurse A to patient – 'you just lie quietly and rest; there's no rush – take your time . . .'

Nurse A, turning to speak to Nurse B – '12 is too many for this type of list – especially when we've more arriving at 1.00. Look, you go to lunch now and then you'll be back to help me see this lot off before we start again . . . do me a favour and see if Mrs Jones is ready to get up and strip her bed before you go . . .'

Nurse A turning back to patient – '. . . feel like a drink yet?'

responsibilities, and therefore feel confident to go home. We must strike the right balance between promoting a return to normality, independence and self-care and mobilizing patients too soon for our own purposes. It is also important to avoid mixed messages. If we want patients to rest for 20 min, then we need to ensure that the environment supports this to the best of our ability; this means turning the radio off and keeping conversations to the minimum. As patients recover and want to sit up, it makes sense to encourage them to engage in conversation with other patients, which in turn will stimulate wakefulness. If the facilities permit, inviting the carer in at this stage will help the patient's recovery. When one patient gets up, the nurse's approach and manner as they assist them is pivotal as other patients are observing the process and can gain or lose confidence as a result. Allow time for patients to sit on the edge of the trolley or bed with their legs down to regain their balance – lie them down again if they feel faint or light headed. Make sure the brakes are on the trolley, that patients have non-slip footwear on and a nurse is with them when they stand up. Have a chair handy; you never know when you might need it.

Reflection Points

Think about how postoperative care is organized in your day unit:

- What aspects of nurse behaviour facilitate or militate against gradual recovery?
- Are any of these amenable to change?
- How might you improve the situation for the patient's benefit?

Promotion of Development and Potential

Preparing for Discharge

Although discharge planning should begin at pre-admission assessment (as discussed in Chapter 5), as the postoperative phase progresses, the focus of nurse activity switches to more explicit discharge preparation, with criteria for discharge being assessed as part of ongoing management (see Table 11.1). Preparation of specific discharge information and effects are collected in readiness for each patient so discharge is as smooth and unrushed as possible; the communication skills of nurses in co-ordinating this information are critical (see Chapter 4).

So what do we mean by discharge criteria in this context? In an early and important piece of work, Stephenson (1990) proposed seven categories to guide decision-making in relation to a patient's readiness for discharge:

- mental state
- mobility
- pain
- eating and drinking
- elimination
- information
- social factors.

Table 11. 1 Postoperative care plan (specimen)

Potential patient problem	Goal/outcome	Nursing actions
Altered conscious level related to anaesthesia/ sedation	Patient is awake, calm orientated and responding lucidly	■ Monitor immediate environment to ensure ongoing safety and orientate patient to surroundings as required ■ Observe skin colour and respiratory rate/pattern for abnormalities ■ Allow adequate time for clearance of anaesthetic/sedative agents prior to discharge *Essential discharge criterion – alert and responsive*
Potential for injury/ side-effects related to anaesthesia/sedation or surgical procedure	Patient remains free of injury Vital signs stable and within normal range	■ Ensure trolley sides are up, brakes are on and call bell is within patient's reach ■ Monitor pulse and B/P in line with individual patient's condition and local protocol ■ Assess any wound dressings ■ Elevate patient's head and assist them in sitting up slowly, providing pillows for support ■ Ambulate gradually taking account of individual patient's abilities *Essential discharge criterion – mobile consistent with pre-operative level and surgical procedure with no dizziness*
Potential for pain	Patient has no pain	■ Observe patient closely for non-verbal indications of pain and act promptly ■ Assist patient in finding comfortable position, providing support for limbs if necessary ■ Use pain assessment tool to evaluate level of discomfort and administer prescribed analgesic ■ Monitor effectiveness of analgesia and discuss with anaesthetist if necessary *Essential discharge criterion – prescribed oral analgesia given and effect evaluated*
Potential for nausea and/or vomiting	Patient has no nausea and able to tolerate oral fluids	■ Avoid sitting patient up rapidly ■ Take account of any pre-operative indications of potential symptoms ■ Provide positive reinforcement and avoid suggestions of nausea ■ Protect patient where possible from nausea-inducing sights and smells ■ Administer prescribed anti-emetic medication prophylactically and evaluate its effect ■ Provide mouthwash as required ■ Provide small amounts of appropriate fluids, increasing as tolerated – avoid fruit juices and coffee *Essential discharge criterion – tolerating oral fluids*

Continued

Table 11. 1 Postoperative care plan (specimen) (*Continued*)

Potential patient problem	Goal/outcome	Nursing actions
Potential deficit in knowledge concerning discharge and ongoing self-care	Patient and carer are able to describe their principal roles and responsibilities of care on return home	■ Avoid where possible patient being given diagnostic information when still under effects of anaesthetic ■ When unavoidable, ensure physician/surgeon is accompanied when they provide post-procedure information so that information can be reinforced prior to discharge ■ Involve identified carer in all pre-discharge assessment and information-giving ■ Assess both patient and carers' understanding of ongoing responsibilities through structured questioning ■ Provide clear, accurate written information to back-up verbal discussion ■ Ensure patient and carer know what to do if problems arise after discharge and have appropriate emergency telephone numbers ■ Invite patient to be included in telephone follow-up service – consent obtained? *Essential discharge criterion – received and understood comprehensive pre-discharge information*

You will see that the nursing actions in relation to the above problems cover the period of time from return from recovery to discharge. You may think that more problems should be documented; that is an individual decision. A second sheet following the same outline would be necessary for documenting other problems identified at postoperative assessment.

Table 11.2 Essential and desirable discharge criteria (adapted from Stephenson 1990)

Category	Essential	Desirable
Mental state	Alert and responsive	Feels clear headed
Mobility	Able to mobilize to pre-operative level within constraints of surgery with no dizziness	
Pain	Has been given appropriate prescribed oral analgesics for pain	No/minimal pain
Eating and drinking	Tolerating oral fluids	Tolerated tea and toast; no nausea or vomiting
Elimination		Passed urine
Information	Verbal explanation of pain management, wound care, driving, alcohol intake, the next 24 h, operation specific information as necessary, whom to contact in an emergency	Written material on same
Social factors	Patient ready to be discharged into care of responsible adult	Further support at home

The factors clearly resemble Orem's six universal health needs and the headings could easily be adapted to suit if so desired (Orem 1991). As a result of a literature review and a descriptive study, Stephenson identified both *essential* and *desirable* criteria in relation to each category (see Table 11.2), providing a useful framework for effective discharge planning. In addition, the essential criteria can be incorporated easily into a standard postoperative care plan.

Other means of assessing readiness for discharge use a scoring system with patients requiring to achieve a minimum score before discharge (Burden 1993).

As indicated earlier in the chapter, opinion is divided as to whether patients should have to pass urine normally before discharge home. In some instances it may be a desirable criterion for discharge from the unit as identified by Stephenson, but for the majority of cases insisting on this can often heighten patient anxiety if they are unable to void and will delay their discharge unnecessarily. Burden (1993) recommends that in order to avoid problems occurring at home, it is advisable that those patients who are in some way predisposed to urinary complications should pass urine spontaneously prior to discharge. She suggests this would include those who have undergone inguinal hernia repair, rectal, urethral or pelvic procedures.

In general, avoiding discharging patients too early usually ensures that any essential criteria are met and discharge protocols must clearly state what such criteria are and who makes the final decision about discharge.

Information Needs for Self-care

With the possible exception of a diagnosis, none of the information provided at this stage in the day surgery process should be new. The questionable practice of surgeons discussing the outcome of surgery and possible future treatment with patients still clearly drowsy from anaesthetic remains an issue of concern and is certainly a source of considerable dissatisfaction for patients (Hawkshaw 1994, Raistrick 1994, Robinson, H. 1994). Nurses must be prepared to take a more active role in ensuring that where such practice cannot be changed, that patients are not seen alone. Uncertainty and anxiety about a diagnosis as a result of postanaesthetic drowsiness will also interfere with the processing of other necessary discharge information.

The responsibilities of both patient and carer for the first 24 h pre-operatively will have been discussed at pre-admission assessment. However, it is essential that the following general principles are reiterated *in the presence of the carer*

- patient must be accompanied home
- patient must have supervision of a responsible adult for the first 24 h
- patient should go home and rest
- patient should not drive, operate machinery or make important decisions or sign anything in the first 24 h.

In addition, procedure-specific information should include:

- drugs – specific instructions regarding prescribed analgesia (see Chapter 8), anti-emetics or antibiotics

- wound care
- when to bathe or shower
- arrangements for dressing renewal and suture removal (if appropriate) – by whom and when
- resuming normal activities
- what to expect – specific symptoms and their duration
- what not to expect and what to do if they occur
- contact telephone numbers for information or in an emergency
- arrangements for follow-up (telephone and outpatients).

It is good practice for a nurse to stay with patients until they actually leave the hospital premises; especially so when the patient needs to wait while their escort collects the car from some distant car park.

Discharge Problems

There will always be occasions when despite comprehensive pre-admission assessment and straightforward anaesthetic and surgery, discharge home is not appropriate. Mostly, these instances are the result of poor control of pain or nausea and vomiting or sometimes as a consequence of difficult surgery. Whatever the cause, *decisions about overnight admission need to be made promptly.* All patients have lives beyond the hospital; children may need picking up from school or other arrangements may need to be made. Whilst there is clearly some mileage in adopting a 'wait and see' approach, leaving both patients and their carers in a state of uncertainty for a couple of hours ultimately achieves little. Rest is difficult, and frequently asking 'how do you feel now?' only serves to make patients feel guilty, as if it is their fault and they really should get up and go home. For an interesting insight into how this feels, we recommend Robinson's (1994) account of his experience of having an arthroscopy.

Patients who wish to go home against medical advice constitute the opposite face of this problem. Historically, patients who dare to disagree with medical opinion have rarely felt supported in their decision, yet the reason for their action may lie with the medical or nursing staff. (This avenue should be explored rather than simply blaming the patient for being irresponsible and feckless.) Despite quite understandable feelings to the contrary, the patient still needs care and it is essential that all attempts are made to persuade them to stay for the recommended period (usually overnight) with the focus on the benefits of doing so. If the patient still insists on going home, then the risks should be clearly and honestly outlined (avoiding exaggerations and inaccuracies) and the patient asked to accept responsibility for their actions through signing a form specifically prepared for the purpose. Two people should be present

Learning Points

- Patients who wish to discharge themselves against medical advice still have a right to quality care.
- A warm and accepting approach may help the patient to re-evaluate their decision.
- Adopting a judgemental and distant approach serves only to reinforce the patient's belief that their decision is the right one (which is probably not the case) and their dissatisfaction with the hospital.

during these discussions and the outcome clearly documented and countersigned in both the care plan and patient's medical notes. A nurse *must* accompany the patient and their carer until they leave the hospital.

Telephone Follow-up Services

Personal experience of a telephone follow-up after inpatient surgery brought home the value of this still-developing service. The purposes of such a service are two-fold:

- to provide post-discharge support for patients, especially when carried out by the patient's primary nurse
- to gather specific data for audit purposes in this early postoperative period (see Chapter 12).

This sounds really supportive and it seems difficult to perceive how an individual would not wish to be contacted to discuss how they are feeling. However, like any other aspect of treatment or care, patients have the right to refuse and permission to contact them at home must be sought prior to discharge. We cannot assume that all patients will have told their families about coming into hospital, and to telephone without consent can constitute a breach of confidentiality; implied consent is not enough. Although the possible consequences of contacting a woman who has undergone termination of pregnancy without obtaining prior consent to do so clearly illustrates this point, the more important principle is that *all patients* have, as Faulder (1985) puts it, '*the right to know and the right to say no*'. Similarly, although an unstructured phone call may seem the best approach to maintain informality, a structured questionnaire should be followed when specific audit data are required. Hawkshaw's (1994) account of a long-term telephone follow-up emphasizes the value of asking about other postoperative side-effects, like interrupted sleep, sore throat, headache, etc. Some dissatisfaction remains with pain relief (especially laparoscopic procedures), privacy, pre-admission information and parking – four Ps for improved patient satisfaction.

Meeting Patient Needs After Discharge

One of the early concerns with increasing day surgery was the potential impact on community services and opinion is still divided on the extent of effects on service provision (Stott 1992). In an investigation into patient satisfaction, Ghosh and Sallam (1994) assessed the level of contact between patients and community services in the first 48 h following surgery. They found the consultation rate (with either general practitioner or district nurse) to be less than 5% with the majority of these being the result of poor pain management.

Some day units are electing to manage any post-discharge services through the appointment of community liaison staff. These services usually focus on those individuals who have undergone intermediate procedures (e.g. hernia repair, laparoscopic sterilization) or specific patient groups (e.g. cataract extractions in the elderly). There are clearly costs associated with developing arrangements such as these, especially as they require experienced and skilled nurses and as yet we have no evidence, beyond anecdotal accounts of increased patient satisfaction, optimized compliance with post-discharge treatments and reduced incidence of complications. This is clearly a subject for investigation.

Informal discussions with day surgery practitioners indicate that there is also an increasing tendency to attach the title 'nurse practitioner' to these posts which can, in itself, be problematic (see Chapter 13). The decision to develop any role such as this must be based on local audit evidence of patient requirements and not on the, as yet, unsupported assertion that no day unit is complete without a 'nurse practitioner'. As Otte (1996) suggests, we must be developing services 'that are designed to meet patients' needs and not purely those of the profession'. Whilst it is very likely that such planned postoperative visits would be welcomed by most patients and may constitute a substantial quality initiative, they must concentrate on particular patient groups and have a specific purpose in order to be cost effective. For example, Drew's (1995) findings indicate that routine postoperative visits to children who had undergone insertion of grommets as day cases are not really necessary. Otte's (1996) study of patients' perceptions of day surgery indicates that patients' satisfaction rests on comprehensive preparation and meticulous discharge planning. Perhaps patient information, nurses' communication skills training and telephone follow-up services are still the areas where time and resources need to be spent in order that *all* patients in day surgery can benefit from a more informed experience. This should include those who have undergone procedures under local anaesthesia; a rapidly growing and diverse patient group.

Discharge arrangements and protocols must therefore achieve a balance between promoting the normality of the day surgery experience (i.e. patients feeling well, minimal or no pain, early resumption of normal activities and return to work) with ensuring that patients have adequate support and know who to contact if things are not right. Experience tells us that generally, patients only contact their general practitioner when they feel unwell or are unsure about some aspect of their recovery; this is especially the case with parents of children who have undergone surgical procedures. The essence of good discharge planning therefore is to ensure that all patients:

- are fit for discharge
- have appropriate analgesia (and anti-emetics if necessary) and know how to take them
- have a clear and realistic knowledge of their recovery period
- are able to recognize abnormal signs and know what to do.

These requirements underline the importance of a rational and comprehensive approach to discharge planning and the communication skills required of nurses in day surgery to ensure that patients well-being is not compromised (as discussed in depth in Chapter 4).

Anecdotal evidence suggests that some patients visit their general practitioner for almost social or courtesy reasons in order to tell them that they have had their operation – especially older patients. After all, it was their doctor who started the process and they should know that it is now complete. It is important to make sure that patients know that their general practitioner will be informed of their surgery and discharge (often that day if the surgery has fax facilities) and they do not need to contact them unless there is a problem.

Summary

The ongoing safety of patients during the postoperative phase of their stay must continue to drive protocols for care and management. Clearly, various approaches are adopted in the organization and delivery of postoperative care across different day surgery units but continuity of care should be the guiding principle. Early recognition of untoward effects of anaesthesia and surgery is easier when the patient is already known to the nurse caring for them. Similarly, prompt and appropriate nursing intervention in the event of postoperative pain or nausea and vomiting is more likely when nurse and patient know each other. This not only improves patient comfort at that time, but their likelihood of straightforward discharge and overall satisfaction with the experience. The postoperative phase is the time when patients initially feel least like going home and their ability to do so depends greatly on the approach of nursing staff and the quality of discharge planning. The time made available to day surgery patients and their carers for their recovery and discharge and the attitudes and skills of the nurses involved in that period are two crucial factors in determining the quality of patient care.

Key Points

- Postoperative management should be organized and delivered in such a way so as to provide the greatest continuity of care for patients.
- There are clear advantages and disadvantages associated with ward and lounge-style second stage recovery areas.
- All postoperative areas require supervision by trained nurses who can recognize the onset of untoward symptoms and initiate appropriate action.
- Decisions to monitor vital signs should be based on the assessment of the effects of anaesthesia on individual patient rather than driven by procedure and tradition.
- Observation is the key to early recognition and treatment of untoward postoperative effects, such as pain or PONV.
- A non-judgemental, accepting approach and patient-centred assessment provides the key to effective pain control.
- Gradual gentle ambulation and introduction of fluids and food help to reduce PONV and therefore improve recovery.
- Early involvement of carers provides valuable support for patients and promotes the perception of returning normality.
- Discharge planning must be based on accepted criteria.
- Problems such as unplanned overnight admission or discharge against medical advice must be dealt with promptly to alleviate distress.
- Telephone follow-up accesses valuable data for audit and changes in practice whilst providing another means of support for patients and their carers.
- Poor pain control is the major reason for patients consulting their general practitioner after discharge; patients must receive appropriate analgesia and all necessary information prior to discharge and know who to contact if problems are experienced.

Recommended reading

Ghosh, S. and Sallam, S. (1994) **Patient satisfaction and postoperative demands on hospital and community services after day surgery.** *British Journal of Surgery* **81**: 1635–1638

Lewin, J. M. E. and Razis, P. A. (1995) **Prescribing practice of take home analgesia for day case surgery.** *British Journal of Nursing* **4**(18): 1047–1051

Otte, D. I. (1996) **Patients' perspectives and experiences of day surgery.** *Journal of Advanced Nursing* **23**: 1228–1237

Robinson, H. (1994) **An unorchestrated encounter – a user's account of day surgery.** *Surgical Nurse* **7**(4): 28–30

References

Burden N. (1993) **Ambulatory Surgery Nursing.** Philadelphia: WB Saunders.

Drew, J. (1995) **Testing the need for a follow-up visit after child day surgery.** *Nursing Standard* **10**(10): 38–43.

Faulder, C. (1985) **Whose body is it?** London: Virago.

Ghosh, S. and Sallam, S. (1994) **Patient satisfaction and postoperative demands on hospital and community services after day surgery.** *British Journal of Surgery* **81**: 1635–1638.

Hawkshaw, D. (1994) **A day surgery patient telephone follow-up survey.** *British Journal of Nursing* **3**(7): 348–350.

Leith, S. E., Hawkshaw, D. and Jackson, I. J. B. (1994) **A national survey of the importance and drug treatment of pain and emesis following surgery.** *Journal Of One-Day Surgery* **4**(2): 24–25.

Medicare Audits Ltd (1993) **The incidence and impact of postoperative nausea and vomiting: Report of a nationwide survey.** Richmond: Synergy Medical Education.

Nightingale, K. (1994) **Postoperative Nausea and Vomiting – Achieving quality of care; a guide for nurses.** Berks: Direct Publishing Solutions.

Ogg, T. W. and Hitchcock, M. (1994) **Day Surgery Post-Operative Nausea and Vomiting.** *Journal of One-Day Surgery* Spring: 18–19.

Orem, D. E. (1991) **Nursing: Concepts of Practice** (Fourth Edition). New York: McGraw-Hill.

Otte, D. I. (1996) **Patients' perspectives and experiences of day surgery.** *Journal of Advanced Nursing* **23**: 1228–1237.

Raistrick, J. (1994) **Day case laparoscopy: patients' views.** *Network* **16**: 8–9.

Ratcliffe, F., Lawson, M. and Millar, J. (1994) **Day-case laparoscopy revisited: have post-operative morbidity and patient acceptance improved?** *Health Trends* **26**(2): 47–49.

Robinson, D. (1993) **Some observations of postoperative nausea and vomiting.** *Journal of One-Day Surgery* Summer: 13–14.

Robinson, H. (1994) **An unorchestrated encounter – A user's account of day surgery.** *Surgical Nurse* **7**(4): 28–30.

Royle, J. A. and Walsh, M. (1992) **Watson's Medical-Surgical Nursing & Related Physiology** (Fourth Edition). London: Baillière Tindall.

Stephenson, M. (1990) **Discharge criteria in day surgery.** *Journal of Advanced Nursing* **15**: 601–613.

Stott, N. C. H. (1992) **Day case surgery generates no increased workload for community based staff. True or false?** *British Medical Journal* **304**: 825–826.

Wilkinson, D., Bristow, A. and Higgins, D. (1992) **Morbidity following day surgery.** *Journal of One-Day Surgery* **2**(1): 5–6.

Chapter 12 Monitoring, standards, audit and quality management

Overview

This chapter is about quality in day surgery. The recurring message for the reader is the requirement for those involved in the health service, and day surgery in particular, to provide their customers with a quality service. The importance of setting of standards that are attainable is considered. The Chapter also introduces the concepts of monitoring, audit and control loops and their place in the management of quality is considered.

Chapter Focus

- The principles of audit
- Monitoring, standards, audit and quality
- Guidance to the selection of suitable performance indicators
- Quality assurance and quality management

Introduction

Audit and subsequent action is of fundamental importance to the successful practice of day surgery. Furthermore, failure to establish standards and implement satisfactory monitoring, audit and quality measures will lead to problems for patients, their general practitioners (GPs) and, ultimately, the day unit concerned.

In Chapter 1, we outlined the history behind the current move to day surgery. This move is occurring rapidly around the UK and indeed is beginning to gain momentum in Europe. It will be achieved by clinicians (surgeons and anaesthetists) transferring inpatient activity to day surgery. Inevitably, this will result in clinicians with little or no experience in day surgery providing this service for the first time. Furthermore, there will be a gradual expansion in the types of operations being performed as day procedures over the next decade. It is important that this clinical activity is monitored and audited to ensure that problems experienced by patients or primary health care colleagues are quickly identified and rectified. The move to day surgery is probably the biggest change in practice in the National Health Service (NHS) over the past decade and requires effective management. If quality is compromised in any way, patients, purchasers of health care, special interest groups and community health councils will soon let us know. So what should we do? What do we mean by monitoring, standards, audit and quality management?

Monitoring

This can be defined as maintaining regular surveillance and can even include the concept of regulation. The combination of surveillance and regulation is useful for our discussion.

Monitoring allows a day unit to judge its performance against explicit standards. Standards in this context can be defined as agreed measures by which performance or achievement can be judged. They can be set locally (by a unit or their purchasers) or nationally (the Patient's Charter) and provide a yardstick against which to measure performance.

Audit

This is a more difficult concept and has caused medical and nursing staff much thought and scratching of heads since its introduction to the NHS! The dictionary is of less help here as it purely reveals the accountancy background of this term with the definition 'official examination of accounts'. In commerce, audit of accounts is undertaken by independent experts who carefully examine part of a company's accounting returns. It would be impossible to examine every detail of a large multinational company's accounts, so only a random part of the accounts undergoes the careful scrutiny of the auditors. Inconsistencies will inevitably lead to the more careful examination of the accounts and may result in the company accounts failing to be approved by the auditors.

This provides an insight into one aspect of audit in the NHS; that is, the careful examination of one area of nursing or medical practice. If we look for the word audit in a thesaurus we find the synonyms *examination, scrutiny, investigation or review.* These provide more of a clue of its meaning in medical practice as each of these can be used in the audit process. The definition taken from the Government's White Paper 'Working for Patients' (DoH 1989), which was largely responsible for the introduction of clinical audit, provides the basis for this Chapter:

> a systematic, critical analysis of the quality of medical care, which includes the procedures used for diagnosis and treatment, the use of resources, and the resulting outcome and quality of life for the patient.

However, there are have been more recent attempts to provide a simpler definition:

> audit is the process of reviewing the delivery of health care to identify deficiencies so that they may be remedied. (Crombie *et al.* 1993)

But this still does not make explicit *who* is delivering health care. The term 'clinical audit' refers to a concept of multidisciplinary audit that crosses multidisciplinary boundaries. Nursing audit is defined by Malby (1995) as

> the systematic evaluation of nursing, resulting in improvements in the quality of care.

Quality

Quality is simply a degree of excellence; a useful but incomplete definition of an essentially subjective experience; what may be felt to represent quality by one individual may be seen as unsatisfactory by another. This is demonstrated in the definition:

> quality is the degree of conformance of all the relevant features and characteristics of the product (or service) to all aspects of a customer's need, limited by the price and delivery he or she will accept. (Groocock 1986)

This has been refined for clinical practice to

quality is a somewhat abstract concept which expresses the capacity of the delivered health care to meet most medical and non-medical goals which are shaped by patients' values and expectations. (Steffen 1988)

Learning Points

- *Monitoring* – maintaining regular surveillance with regulation.
- *Standards* – an agreed measure by which performance or achievement can be judged.
- *Audit* – a systematic, critical analysis of the quality of clinical care, which includes the procedures used for diagnosis and treatment, the use of resources and the resulting outcome for the patient.
- *Quality* – a somewhat abstract concept which expresses the capacity of the delivered health care to meet most medical and non-medical goals which are shaped by patients' values and expectations.

Monitoring

Having defined what monitoring is, it is important to identify *what* should be monitored. The first and easy answer is that any standards that have been set should be monitored. Much of the monitoring in this Chapter has to do with the organization and running of a day unit but later monitoring in relation to standards is explored.

Managers clearly require information that is both accurate and timely to run an efficient service; information that is inaccurate can lead to misjudgements. It may lead to inappropriate counselling of clinical colleagues or indeed the inaccuracy of the data may be demonstrated during discussions following which it will be difficult to regain the faith of managers or clinicians in the value of future data. Timely information is important as this allows managers to identify problems at an early stage and deal with them quickly. One example would be the production of a monthly report about the patients who 'did not attend' (DNAs) for their operation. If the monthly DNA rate revealed a problem in one specialty then this can be examined and corrective action taken. However, a report published on a 6-monthly or yearly basis would lead to unnecessary delays. Therefore, monitoring must take account of report design and frequency as well as content. Box 12.1 lists some factors that a unit may consider monitoring.

Box 12.1 Factors suitable for monitoring

- Number of cancellations as a result of the patient being found to be unsuitable on the day of surgery
- Proportion of patients admitted overnight by surgeons
- Proportion of patients readmitted within 1 week
- Proportion of patients who did not attend
- Utilization of theatre time by each surgeon
- Proportion of day case procedures in hospital done in the day unit
- Proportion of day surgery to elective inpatient surgery
- Number of patients contacting the unit post-discharge with problems
- Number of patients requiring intervention of GP post-discharge
- Number of patients cancelled on day of operation
- Number of patients waiting longer than 18 months for their operation

The last two factors in Box 12.1 form part of the Patient's Charter and must be monitored but most can be seen to be essential for the efficient management of a day unit. It should be clear why this kind of information is necessary; consider each in turn before continuing with this Chapter.

The number of cancellations on the day of surgery provides a clear indication of the effectiveness of the pre-admission assessment service. The proportion of patients admitted overnight provides early warning of problem areas that need attention. The reasons for all admissions should be carefully examined. Are patients being assessed appropriately or are appropriate operations being performed on the unit? Similarly, the number of patients re-admitted due to complications of their surgery is important – is the surgeon operating on inappropriate patients? Every time a patient does not attend the opportunity is lost to use a valuable resource, that is, the nursing and clinical time that has been set aside for the management of that patient. We can no longer be complacent about missing patients; it is important to identify problem areas and attempt to rectify the problem.

Utilization of theatres (over and under) is again a difficult problem to discuss with surgeons; however, it must be tackled and accurate information is vital. The proportion of day cases performed in the day unit and the overall proportion of day procedures compared to numbers of elective surgical procedures provide an indication of the effectiveness of the policy of the hospital. These are figures that purchasers will ask for. The number of patients contacting the unit with problems or requiring intervention of their GP post-discharge provides an indication of problems with patient selection, anaesthetic technique, surgical technique or discharge arrangements.

These are some of the reasons that you may consider monitoring some of these areas; indeed, you may well have thought of others that are more important for your unit. It is important to remember that the above data will incur costs for its collection and storage so it is important to be clear about the information that is necessary for the management of your service.

Learning Point

Monitoring should provide information that is:

- relevant
- accurate
- timely
- appropriate
- clear
- complete.

Standards

The next area that requires consideration is the setting and monitoring of standards. In fact the last two areas covered in Box 12.1 refer to national standards set in the Patient's Charter by which our performance can be judged. The only other national standards that have to be monitored and provided are for the new league tables produced by the government in which day surgery rates (as a percentage of elective inpatient activity for certain operations) are compared. Standards may also be imposed locally by the purchasers, for example GP fundholders or health authorities. The majority of standards that may be used by a day unit are produced as part of the management monitoring already mentioned or as part of quality initiatives from within the unit. The parameters in Box 12.1 lend themselves to the setting of standards; for example a unit may decide that the utilization of scheduled theatre time should be greater than 85%, or less than 1% of patients should be found to be unsuitable for surgery on admission. Standards should be set so that the staff who will work to them feel that they are:

- *equitable* – staff feel they are all working to similar targets
- *essential* – the targets are linked to a goal that is very important
- *attainable* – staff should feel they have a good chance of meeting the standard
- *adjustable* – there must be the ability to change the standard if its has truly been set too high
- *inviolable* – meeting the standard will not result in it automatically being made harder in the future.

Standards can be incorporated into the quality specifications laid down in contracts for day surgery. Donaldson (1994) identifies such quality clauses as one of the ways in which purchasers are actively attempting to raise standards and improve patient outcomes, but also suggests that the extent to which such action is appropriate is open to debate.

It would be wrong to talk about standards without considering the subject of *control*. Having established standards, it is important to measure performance (i.e. monitor), compare this to the standard and then decide if corrective action is needed. This process is known as a *control loop* and the steps involved are shown in Fig. 12.1.

It should be noted that when performance does not achieve the standard this control loop allows the options of taking action to improve performance, to continue without change and, importantly, to revise the standard if it has been set too high. Having explored standards and control loops, it is appropriate now to consider audit, where it will be seen that both these concepts have a part to play.

Figure 12.1 A control loop

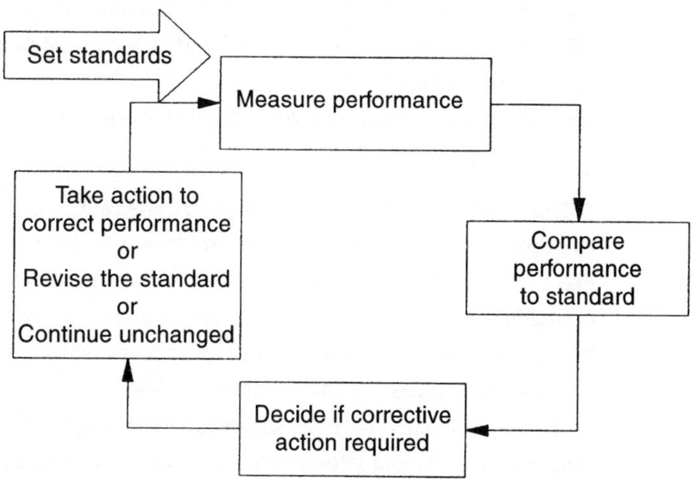

Audit

Usually questions asked about audit are:

- What is audit?
- Why do we do it?
- How should we do it?

We have already defined what audit is and we will consider methods of audit under the last question. However, it is again worth considering *why* we should do it. The simple answer is that it is expected since the publication of the White Paper 'Working for Patients' (DoH 1989). However, this forms only part of the answer. Nursing and clinical practice is moving forward at an accelerating pace and until the massive investment in audit by the NHS this was largely occurring on an *ad hoc* basis. Clearly, medical and nursing practice for the management of illness differs across the world, between countries, between regions, between hospitals and even between clinicians and nursing staff in the same hospital. Who is right? Which method achieves the best outcomes? These are questions we can no longer ignore in the cash-limited health services in which we have to work. Audit forms one of the processes that allows for serious consideration of the management of patients and can be used to:

- to promote change
- to increase effectiveness and/or efficiency
- to increase job satisfaction
- to identify training and professional needs
- to address legal implications
- for contracting requirements
- to identify and disseminate 'good practice'
- to improve teamwork
- to improve communication.

Crombie *et al.* (1993) offer a useful and alternative way of clarifying the use of audit, linking it to health care delivery's 'three Es':

- efficacy – concerned with whether treatment works – requires clinical research
- effectiveness – concerned with whether such treatments work in practice – this is the realm of clinical audit
- efficiency – concerned with whether resources are being used effectively – uses health economics techniques.

This brings us to *how* we should do it. Classically, audit is linked to a process called the *audit cycle* which is very similar to the control loop introduced earlier in the Chapter as can be seen in Fig. 12.2. The important feature is that it is indeed a loop and following one turn of the cycle and having instigated changes it is important to follow the cycle again to see if the changes have had the desired effect. The cycle is useful for staff attempting to start an audit project but there are a couple of 'grey areas' that need to be considered.

The first problem is deciding what to audit; that is, the areas of current practice you are going to observe and set standards for. The earlier discussion about setting of standards should help here. It is

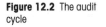

Figure 12.2 The audit cycle

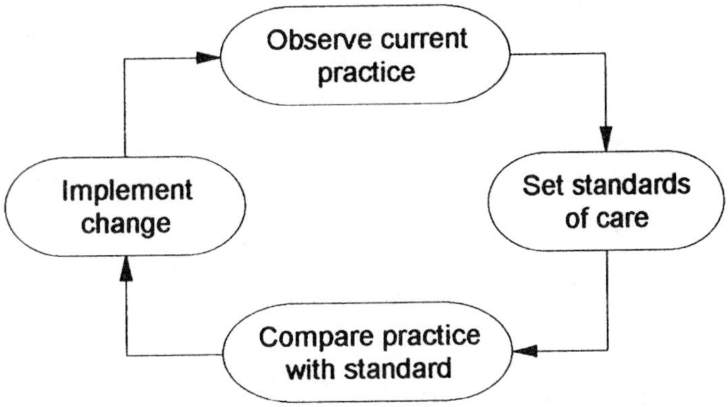

important to consider each of the following five headings suggested; that is, are they equitable, essential, attainable, adjustable and inviolate. The next problem is when to stop the cycle – that is, at what stage does the collection of data and regular review become a process of considering routine data? Routine data collection holds no audit value – although it may well provide positive, morale-boosting feedback for staff. These questions must be asked by the individuals performing the audit task. Unless the project reveals the requirement for further significant improvement, in practice the team should consider moving to another project after using the cycle twice.

Quality

Quality is an elusive target that commercial companies and the health service is being pressurized to chase. It would be foolish and somewhat naive to believe that this push for quality is only coming from senior management in our organizations. Indeed the Patient's Charter is frequently *blamed* in health circles for the massive increase in complaints that we have seen over the past few years. But this massive increase should not be surprising – patients are being promised improved standards of care, respect for their privacy, dignity and cultural and spiritual beliefs *and* shorter waiting lists (Dixon 1994). Consumerism is on the increase and the Patient's Charter may well just be political recognition of this fact – a cynic might even suggest that it represents an attempt to gain Brownie points from the electorate!

When presented with what we believe to be 'shoddy' goods or service we are all more likely to complain, rather than use the 'grin and bear it' attitude of previous generations. This is not to say that consumerism is only present in the younger generations; this new found freedom is enjoyed and fully used by all ages! In considering these issues and the concept of quality we should remember this freedom actually represents a major step forward for us all as consumers. If this important fact is kept in mind it will help us all maintain the all-important positive attitude to the management of quality.

We have already defined quality as a somewhat abstract concept which expresses the capacity of the delivered health care to meet most medical and non-medical goals which are shaped by patients' values and expectations. Now it is important to consider *why* is it needed. A wise man once said 'the attention to detail is what separates the truly great from those who are merely adequate'. Quality is important to patients and to staff in the health service, but it is also important because it can reduce costs and provide an even better service to patients. One of the fundamental aims in the health service is to care for patients and the majority of staff have a real commitment to care for people. Where nursing and medical staff work in a service that is *not* providing quality care they can become demoralized, demotivated and frustrated. Effort expended in rectifying this situation, helping staff identify problems and supporting them in their plans to rectify these, can lead to increased job satisfaction, motivation and morale as well as provide the quality the patients have every right to expect. *Quality therefore has to be about change.*

It is important to remember that quality includes cost – the cost the consumer is willing to pay for that service. In the health service this cost, measured as long waiting times and overall poor service, has traditionally been high; for example large numbers of patients sent the same clinic time to ensure there were no gaps due to patients not attending or being seen more quickly than expected. However, patients were willing to 'pay' this cost as it was seen to be a necessary part of the NHS. However, the situation has now changed and this cost is seen as being too high. When considering quality, it is important to remember that no matter how good the quality of the service we supply in our area is, it is only as strong as its weakest point.

Consider a patient and carer that have been well looked after by nursing and medical staff. The patient is discharged armed with all the necessary information and analgesia and the operation has been a complete success. When they get to the front door the carer's car has been clamped and it takes 20 min to find someone to unclamp it. The porter during this process proceeds to lecture the carer about where to park at the hospital, a situation made worse by the fact that the area where the carer should have parked was already full when they arrived! Does this sound familiar? How would you feel? Would you wish to return to that hospital? This point was neatly captured by a senior executive in British Airways who said 'a service industry is vulnerable at its weakest point. If you go to a restaurant the food can be magnificent but if the service is lousy the chances are you will never go back again. That's the crux of it' (G. Cuthbert)

Quality Issues for Patients

Before we look at day surgery as a specific area let us consider what is important to customers. An extremely useful study by Berry *et al.* (1985) based on in-depth interviews of customers found that their assessment of quality can be summarized into 10 factors. It is useful to consider each of these with examples of good and bad practice (Table 12.1). These factors should make sense to all of us as consumers and indeed none is irrelevant to our practice.

Patients in hospital are often anxious, stressed and frightened (no less so in day surgery) and staff should be doing all they to can to lessen these feelings by providing adequate facilities, information (e.g. at pre-admission assessment) and ensuring they are provided with appropriate support and treated without undue delay. Some obvious quality areas in day surgery for patients include:

- *General factors:*
  ease of parking
  ease of finding the ward
  absence of long wait at reception
  appearance of surroundings
  level of privacy on the ward
  atmosphere on the ward.

Table 12.1 Customer assessment of quality

Factors	Good practice	Bad practice
Reliability	Punctual arrival of train	Failure to phone customer back as agreed
Responsiveness	Maintenance staff who service equipment at short notice	Long queues
Competence	Staff carry out task with skill and competence	Bank fails to cancel standing order then charges fee for resulting overdraft
Access	Easy to find one's way. Easy to get to	Poor signposting. Limited car parking
Courtesy	Polite and helpful staff	Senior staff patronizing and condescending
Communication	Medical staff who explain the diagnosis and alternative forms of treatment without using jargon	Lack of information when trains are delayed as to the cause and duration of the delay
Credibility	A solicitor you feel you can trust and depend on	A used-car salesman who uses hard-sell tactics
Security	A feeling of personal safety and confidentiality	Unlit access at night
Understanding/knowing the customer	Staff who make an effort to meet a customer's individual requirements	Staff who do not recognize a regular customer
Tangibles	Pleasing physical appearance of facilities and staff	Poor or out-of-date equipment being used for the service

- *Nursing factors:*
  appearance and manner of nurses, especially that all-important first contact
  accurate and appropriate information about what is going to happen at each stage of the admission
  inclusion of carer or relative
  attention to individual concerns.
- *Medical factors:*
  the appearance and manner of the medical staff
  the clarity of the explanation provided about the procedure
  after-effects of anaesthetic
  the success of the procedure
  complications occurring at home.

These lists are by no means exhaustive but provide a framework on to which we can add those issues felt to be important locally. Compare these headings with the 10 factors in Table 12.1 and consider how you might address those we have failed to cover.

Assessment of Quality in Day Surgery

Owing to the pioneering work of the Audit Commission, we have a useful tool for the assessment of the quality of service we are supplying to patients. The Commission asked the Health Services Research Unit of the London School of Hygiene and Tropical Medicine to develop and validate a questionnaire for patients (Audit Commission, 1991). Computer software for the analysis of the large amount of data recorded by these questionnaires was also developed. Despite some initial teething problems with the analysis software this questiionnairehas been used extensively across the UK and offers the opportunity for comparison of performance between units. We recommend that if you have not used or seen this questionnaire that you find the above Audit Commission reference. This contains a full copy of the questionnaire and details about its development, how to use it and the results of its use in field trials in three health authorities. Data from this questionnaire consistently identify what we refer to as the '*three Ps of patient satisfaction*' (or more accurately, *dissatisfaction*):

- pain
- privacy
- parking.

The first two of these factors are clearly amenable to quality improvement; the third, as suggested in the earlier example, is more dependent on available space and the goodwill of parking attendants. On a smaller scale, Buttery *et al.* (1993) identified the following areas for improvement:

- pre-operative waiting (felt to be too long – think about anxiety rising during this time – Chapter 7)
- recovery area uncomfortable and lacking in privacy (how would you feel about discussing your periods or being sick in front of strangers? – Chapters 7 & 11)
- more information regarding feeling 'groggy' (brings us back to realistic expectations and the need for clear accurate information – Chapter 5)
- something more substantial to eat when recovered (difficult to predict need – Chapter 11)

Quality Management

No discussion on quality would be complete without reference to quality management and *total quality management* (TQM) in particular. There are other terms that you will come across when reading about this area such as *quality control* and *quality assurance*. Again, it is important that we start by considering what is meant by these terms.

Quality control is controlling and monitoring the process to produce quality products and services. Quality assurance is the prevention of quality problems through planned and systematic activities including documentation, training and reviewing the process. Quality management is the management philosophy which applies to all parts of the organization, involving managing all functions and activities to achieve quality.

Learning Points

- ***Quality control*** is controlling and monitoring the process to produce quality products and services.
- ***Quality assurance*** is the prevention of quality problems through planned and systematic activities including documentation, training and reviewing the process.
- ***Quality management*** is the management philosophy which applies to all parts of the organization, involving managing all functions and activities to achieve quality.

Several names are linked to quality management and TQM in particular, the most notable perhaps being W. E. Deming and Philip Crosby. It is interesting to note that Deming, who was American, had to go to Japan to gain an audience for his ideas in the 1950s. His influence has certainly played a part in the success of Japanese industry since that time. Crosby promotes an approach to quality based on what he terms *zero defects* (Crosby 1984). In other words, organizations should not be happy that 90% of their customers are satisfied as this translates to them being content that 10% are dissatisfied with their service or product. Crosby argues that successful organizations cannot and should not accept this attitude. Only 0% dissatisfaction will do, which sounds rather idealistic and unattainable. However, the attitude that quality is *worth* continually striving for, is the key issue here and one that is relevant to the context of day surgery and patient satisfaction.

Summary

In health care terms, the drive to improve quality of care has tended to focus on current and politically sensitive initiatives such as the reduction of waiting lists, increasing patient involvement in care and improving the physical environment for patients and their families. These are clearly important quality concerns in day surgery. However, as Sheldon (1994) points out:

> At the heart of quality must be the effectiveness and cost effectiveness of interventions. Without ensuring that health technologies are effective and are delivered appropriately then many of the other dimensions of quality may simply be window dressing.

The rising tide of consumerism is being felt by all who work in the health service. There are many reasons for this and though the Patient's Charter may well be adding to these it is not the cause of this very real swell of public opinion.

Attention to quality through the use of standards and monitoring are some of the skills we need to develop within the health service to contain this problem.

Key Points

- Monitoring describes the process of maintaining regular surveillance with regulation.
- Standards are an agreed measure by which performance or achievement can be judged.
- Audit is a systematic, critical analysis of the quality of clinical care, which includes the procedures used for diagnosis and treatment, the use of resources and the resulting outcome for the patient.
- Quality is a somewhat abstract concept which expresses the capacity of the delivered health care to meet most medical and non-medical goals which are shaped by patients' values and expectations.
- Monitoring should provide information that is relevant, accurate, timely, appropriate, clear and complete.

- Standards should be equitable, essential, attainable, adjustable and inviolable.
- Quality control is controlling and monitoring the process to produce quality products and services.
- Quality assurance is the prevention of quality problems through planned and systematic activities including documentation, training and reviewing the process.
- Quality management is the management philosophy which applies to all parts of the organization, involving managing all functions and activities to achieve quality.

Recommended Reading

Audit Commission (1992) **Making time for patients. A handbook for ward sisters.** London: HMSO

Jones, A. and McDonnell, U. (1993) **Managing the Clinical Resource. An action guide for health care professionals.** London: Baillière Tindall

Sale, D. (1990) Quality Assurance – **Essentials of nursing management.** Hong Kong: Macmillan

Snowley, G. D., Nicklin, P. J. and Birch, J. A. (1992) **Objectives for Care – Specifying standards for clinical nursing** (Second Edition). London: Wolfe
All texts provide further perspectives and information on standards and quality issues in health care

Audit Commission (1991) **NHS Occasional Papers. Measuring quality: The patient's view of day surgery.** London: HMSO
We strongly suggest that all staff familiarize themselves with the issues covered in this key document and the areas covered by the patient questionnaire

Closs, S. J. and Cheater, F. M. (1996) **Audit or research – what is the difference?** *Journal of Clinical Nursing* **5**: 249–256
A useful article explaining the differences and similarities between research and audit

References

Audit Commission (1991) **NHS Occasional Papers. Measuring quality: The patient's view of day surgery.** London: HMSO.

Berry, L., Zeithami, V. and Parasuraman, A. (1985) **A Practical Approach to Quality.** Joiner Associates Inc.

Buttery, Y., Sissons, J. and Williams, N. (1993) **Patients' views one week after day surgery with general anaesthesia.** *Journal of One-Day Surgery* Summer: 6–8.

Crombie, I. K., Davies, H. T. O., Abraham, S. C. S. and du V. Florey, C. (1993) **The Audit Handbook.** Chichester: John Wiley.

Crosby, P. B. (1984) **Quality Without Tears.** London: McGraw-Hill.

Department of Health (1989) **Working for patients.** London: HMSO.

Dixon, E. (1994) **The Patients Charter – its implications for surgery.** *British Journal of Theatre Nursing* **4**(4): 19–22.

Donaldson, L. (1994) **Building quality into contracting and purchasing.** *Quality Health Care* **3**(supplement): 37–40.

Groocock, J. M. (1986) **The Chain of Quality.** London: Wiley.

Malby, R. (Ed) (1995) **Clinical Audit for Nurses and Therapists.** London: Scutari.

Sheldon, T. A. (1994) **Quality: link with effectiveness.** *Quality Health Care* **3**(supplement): 41–45.

Steffen, G. F. (1988) **Quality medical care: a definition.** *Journal of the American Medical Association* **260**: 56.

Chapter 13 Future trends in day surgery

Overview

This chapter could have had many titles, for example, 'gazing in the ether' or 'consulting the runes'. Indeed, it may prove to be less accurate than the weather forecast in the UK! What we provide here are simply our views and opinions of what the future might hold for the specialty. We hope that it promotes thought and discussion of some of the problems currently facing the National Health Service (NHS) and some of the developments possibly occurring in the next 10 years.

Chapter Focus

- Free-standing day surgery units
- Children's services
- Hotel services
- Minimally invasive surgery
- Developments in anaesthesia
- Issues for medical staffing
- Issues for nursing and professional practice

Introduction

There are many variables that will effect progress both in the health service as a whole and in the field of day surgery. External influences such as politics and the creed of the government in power over the next 5–10 years will undoubtedly play a major role. However, this will not be the only influence. Increasing costs of medical technology and the increasing expertise of medical and nursing staff in managing previously incurable conditions will also lay a financial burden on the service. This will be compounded by the increasing numbers of elderly people in the population.

Medical technology will doubtlessly continue to move forward, particularly in the surgical specialties leading to new procedures many of which may be included under the heading of *minimally invasive surgery*. Indeed, more procedures may come under the increasing skills of interventional radiologists, particularly in the field of vascular surgery.

Some indication of our future direction can be gained from the USA where, as explained in Chapter 1, day surgery has developed at a greater pace. Certain issues or techniques of management that are already being pursued both in the USA and in this country will increasingly have an influence over the next decade.

Free-standing Day Surgery Units

These are now commonplace in the USA with over 1200 units in existence. As explained in Chapter 1, these have been developed in response to the desire to minimize the costs of the common procedures performed in these units. The cost of these procedures in a free-standing day surgery unit in the USA are less than in a major hospital due to the reduced overheads (indirect costs) as explained in Chapter 2. In the UK, day surgery units including most of the few current free-standing units are part of a provider unit, that is an NHS Trust hospital, and therefore share the overheads of the whole organization. However, there may yet be room for a change in this situation.

There are now some general practitioner (GP) fundholders in the UK who are considering or are currently providing day surgery facilities from their premises. This may well have an effect on the costing of day surgery procedures. However, developments along these lines, whether in local 'cottage' hospitals or specially-built GP surgeries, will depend on several factors. The principal factors will include medical manpower, safety aspects, economics and, naturally, the politics of the government in power. Medical staffing is discussed later in this chapter but it is worth noting now that there are already shortages of certain specialists. This shortage of specialists and the current reduction in junior doctors' hours would lead to a problem in provision of services at more peripheral sites. It is interesting to note that a trend in this direction would not be something completely new, it would merely be moving back in time to how many services were provided in the 1950s and 1960s in local hospitals (the only difference being that previously it was inpatient surgery).

Safety aspects are already being considered by many specialist bodies. The Association of Anaesthetists in a recent document titled 'Surgery and General Anaesthesia in General Practitioner Premises' covered this topic carefully. It fully describes the requirements for premises, equipment, support staff and the levels of expertise required. The important aspect, however, is the recognition that it is possible to provide anaesthetic services outside our main hospitals.

However, economics and political will are (along with the manpower issue) the major determinants that will direct this path of development. Economically, although these services could be provided in free-standing units with lower overheads and therefore at a lower cost to the purchaser, there remains one large problem. Currently, these day surgery patients *contribute to the overheads* of the large hospitals – removal of these cases and their contribution would automatically increase the cost of the provision of all other services within that hospital. Therefore, in this scenario there may be no financial gain in moving to free-standing units. It is important to remember, however, that there may well be gains *as perceived by the consumer* by bringing the service closer to their community.

It should be apparent from this perhaps simplistic view on this potential area of development that the setting up of a free-standing day surgery unit by a third party (private company or a Trust) in another hospital's catchment area could have a devastating effect on its viability.

Children's Day Surgery Units

One major aspect of day surgery in many units is the provision of services for children which, as in any setting, requires clear and unambiguous standards of care. Thornes (1991), in the National

Box 13.1 Standards for care of children as day cases

1. The admission is planned in an integrated way to include pre-admission, day of admission and post-admission care, and to incorporate the concept of a planned transfer of care to primary and/or community services.
2. The child and parent are offered preparation both before and during the day of admission.
3. Specific written information is provided to ensure that parents understand their responsibilities throughout the episode.
4. The child is admitted to an area designated for day cases and not mixed with acutely ill inpatients.
5. The child is neither admitted nor treated alongside adults.
6. The child is cared for by identified staff specifically designated to the day-case area.
7. Medical, nursing and all other staff are trained for, and skilled in, work for children and their families, in addition to the expertise needed for day-case work.
8. The organization and delivery of patient care are planned specifically for day cases so that every child is likely to be discharged within the day.
9. The building, equipment and furnishings comply with safety standards for children.
10. The environment is homely and includes areas for play and other activities designed for children and young people.
11. Essential documentation, including communication with the primary and/or community services, is completed before each child goes home so that after-care and follow-up consultations are not delayed.
12. Once care has been transferred to the home, nursing support is provided, at a doctor's request, by nurses trained in the care of sick children.

Association for the Welfare of Children in Hospital document 'Caring for Children in the Health Services', proposes 12 quality standards for a planned package of care for children (0–16 years) admitted as day cases; these are listed in Box 13.1.

Although these standards give a clear indication of what should be achieved, it is also evident that the practices of many day surgery units are very different – yet they would argue that children receive high quality care. In the light of the Allitt Inquiry (1994) and the Department of Health's (1991) recommendations, day surgery provision must take account of the differing needs of children. In some ways the Allitt Inquiry achieved more for children's nurses than children themselves as the skills and experience and overall position of registered sick children's nurses (RSCNs) has been strengthened as a result. The Department of Health (DoH) strongly advise that provider hospitals take account of the above standards in their consultations with purchasers. In order to meet these standards, the DoH suggests that Trusts have four options:

- creation of a discrete children's day unit, staffed by appropriately qualified and experienced nurses
- use of a planned designated area in a children's inpatient ward
- designation of a separate children's area in a day surgery unit
- planned, designated 'children's days'; e.g. once a week.

Choice depends largely on local demand for children's day surgery, as the costs of the first option are clearly high, but there is little doubt that it is the best option as children are best cared for by nursing staff who are experienced and qualified in meeting their needs. However, many Trusts do not have that level of demand and, consequently, one of the other options is utilized. When children are cared for on an adult day surgery unit, the DoH (1991) advise that an RSCN is available 24 h a day to advise on nursing care. Nurses on day surgery units cannot afford complacency or protectionism about the children in their care and close liaison with the hospital's paediatric unit is essential. The employment of RSCNs in the community must also be seen as a sound investment.

Hotel Services

It is important to be clear about what is meant by the provision of hotel services or a patient hotel. In this discussion we refer to the provision of accommodation on or near a hospital site that can be used by a patient following discharge from the hospital. It would be staffed by receptionist staff and would not employ nursing staff. The service would provide a bedroom (suitable for patient and a carer – this is especially important for children) with *en suite* facilities. There should be dining, kitchen and sitting areas for the 'guests' and meals should be provided. Stay in the hotel should be limited to a maximum period of somewhere between 2 and 5 days.

At first it may seem difficult to understand how such a facility may help in day surgery. The commonest reasons for refusing a patient for day surgery are social reasons – lack of easy availability of a telephone, toilet or even a carer. The provision of hotel facilities can circumvent many of these, therefore allowing us to increase the number of patients treated. Furthermore, if the hotel is located on the hospital site it offers several advantages for other patient groups. Potentially, those cataract patients who are reviewed the morning following their surgery could use this facility to save having to travel back to the hospital from home. Surgeons may be encouraged to attempt larger or different procedures on patients as a day case if they knew they were staying on the hospital site and could be transferred back to the hospital quickly should a problem occur. Operations such as laparoscopic cholecystectomy, bilateral varicose vein surgery, adenoidectomy or even tonsillectomy may be included in this list by some clinicians. Economics once again form the backbone of the move to the provision of hotel beds. As they are staffed purely by a small number of non-nursing personnel, they cost much less to run.

Minimally Invasive Surgery

Minimally invasive surgery has undergone a somewhat painful gestation period in the UK. It was unfortunately seen as a necessary development for every hospital and indeed almost every surgeon across the UK. As indicated in Chapter 5, essentially experimental techniques being carried out by skilled enthusiasts were rapidly extended to the rest of the NHS with little or no control before their role and effectiveness had been fully evaluated (Bloor & Maynard 1994). Whilst some doctors remain 'reluctant to countenance evaluation of techniques which they feel are unambiguously beneficial' (Baggott 1994), valuable lessons have been learned by surgeons, Trusts and the NHS Executive (NHSE) from this scenario and hopefully similar problems will not occur in the future.

We now have several recognized training hospitals throughout the UK who receive national funding to provide training in minimally invasive surgery. These centres will also help co-ordinate the development of this service and its careful evaluation. There can be little doubt that we shall see subspecialization in surgical specialties and a general move away from the 'generalist' who would attempt any operation. There will be specialists in the techniques of minimally invasive surgery in each major hospital. These specialists will gradually increase the number of procedures that can be done using these techniques. Already, laparoscopic cholecystectomy is being performed as a day surgery procedure in some units across the UK, though this is more common in the USA. Laparoscopic hernia repairs are likewise common, but are lengthier procedures and have yet to prove their long-term efficacy, in terms of recurrence (Philips 1994). Minimally invasive surgery will reduce the lengths of stay of patients for the surgical population but there will be limits to which procedures can be carried out on a day surgery basis. As Phillips (1994) points out, there is a considerable increase in operating time that has to be taken account of in allocation of resources. However, the use of these techniques along with hotel or low dependency facilities is a strong possibility for the future.

Developments in Anaesthesia

There have already been some major advances in anaesthesia that have influenced the move to day surgery over the past decade. The availability of anaesthetic agents that are removed from the body more quickly has been of major benefit to patients. The induction agent propofol and the new volatile agent sevoflurane are two examples of these drugs. Propofol has offered the anaesthetist the opportunity to use what is termed as total intravenous anaesthesia (TIVA). Within this type of anaesthetic the anaesthetist does not use any nitrous oxide or volatile agents to keep the patient anaesthetized. The patient breathes (or is ventilated with) an oxygen/air mixture and anaesthesia is maintained by using infusions of propofol and possibly an analgesic agent. This technique offers obvious advantages for the avoidance of atmospheric pollution with nitrous oxide and the volatile agents. However, there is evidence that it may also contribute to a low incidence of postoperative nausea and vomiting, which is useful in day surgery. Further developments that will be seen in this area will include the availability of increasingly sophisticated computer controlled infusion pumps. The next generation of these now becoming available includes the facility to program the patient's age, body weight and the desired blood level of the agent. The computer then controls the pump to achieve these levels. The measurement of level of anaesthesia (i.e. how deeply the patient is anaesthetized) has been a major goal of research in anaesthesia for some years. In the next few years we will see the availability of monitors for this purpose which can then be linked to our infusion devices to help control the actual blood level of the agent required for each individual patient. These developments will increase the safety in anaesthesia and ensure that patients receive enough anaesthetic agent so they do not remember their operation. More importantly, they will ensure that patients do not receive more than is necessary of the anaesthetic agent and therefore aid their recovery process. Similar links as described above can be made with the control of the new volatile agents such as sevoflurane.

The scarcity of anaesthetists may well lead to a further rise in the popularity of local anaesthetic techniques. Already, many surgeons have become very skilful in the application of nerve blocks because of this problem. This is true of gynaecologists, who can perform many procedures including hysteroscopy under local anaesthesia; plastic surgeons; and orthopaedic surgeons, who undertake quite major surgery on the upper or lower limb using nerve blocks. Hernias and cataract extraction are two procedures where the use of local anaesthesia may offer some advantages over general anaesthesia. However, this move to try and circumvent the anaesthetic shortage leaves a problem of what is termed the operator/anaesthetist. For some procedures, the use of an operator anaesthetist is discouraged by the Royal Colleges. The best example of this is for cataract surgery (Royal College of Anaesthetists and the College of Ophthalmologists 1993). This report recommends that an anaesthetist should be present to monitor the patient and in order to give resuscitation, should it be required.

Theatres are already training paramedics, nursing and operating department assistants in advanced life support (ALS) techniques. Individuals who complete these courses are working in an area that can provide the practice necessary to maintain these skills. The appropriateness of using an expensive and rare resource in an area that *could* potentially be managed by suitably trained staff will be seriously questioned by Trusts in the UK. This could well lead to a change in the training needs for the various theatre personnel in day surgery units. The National Vocational Qualification (NVQ) in Operating Department Practice (level 3) is proving popular with theatre managers for both nurses and operating department assistants (ODAs). Hence operating department or theatre practitioners will have varied experience and backgrounds but the resulting skill (and salary) mix may prove economically attractive for Trusts. It is also quite likely that nurses 'fast tracking' through this programme are doing so as there is a dearth of nursing courses that offer the required technical skills. Although nurse education has a clear role in developing courses to meet changing needs, nursing as a profession must decide what nursing is actually about. This concern leads us on to consider medical and nursing staffing issues in general and how they might impact upon future developments in day surgery.

Issues in Medical Staffing

There are several potential problem areas that need to be considered when discussing medical staffing. The first fact is that there is currently a shortage of suitable applicants for consultant posts in several specialties in the UK. For the purposes of our discussion the relevant shortage specialties include some of the smaller surgical specialties (e.g. urology), but most importantly there is a large shortage of anaesthetists in the UK. This has caused many problems for hospitals around the country. In the face of a shortage it is important to use the staff in post to their optimal potential and therefore avoid expansion into any less productive area, for example provision of anaesthetic services to a peripheral unit. This shortage we are assured is merely temporary but recruitment will remain a problem for many hospitals for some time to come. Further pressure on medical staff comes from the demands of the reduction in junior doctors hours (NHS ME 1991) This reduction in hours has been achieved by:

- making the people on call work harder by covering larger areas
- employing intermediate grade doctors to help with the on call work
- appointing new consultant posts to release junior doctors
- employment of more support staff – phlebotomists, clerks
- extension of the nurse's role – administration of intravenous drugs, establishing intravenous access, etc; in itself a contentious issue – see later in this chapter.

However, the fundamental point is that a large number of work hours have been lost from hospitals. This cannot occur without a change in the service and, despite the initiatives mentioned above, many departments are finding it increasingly difficult to maintain current levels of activity. Specialties that provide a service, such as radiology, pathology and anaesthesia, have suffered most of these difficulties. The appointment of new surgeons and physicians on the basis of reducing junior doctor workload inevitably leads to more work and more patients being treated. As well as putting added strain on these service departments it puts an added strain on nursing, physiotherapy and other services. However, the difficulties faced in medical staffing have a further twist – the Calman Report (Working Group on Specialist Medical Training 1993). This deals with bringing the education of doctors into line with European models. The reasons for the development of this report are complex and involve a requirement to conform with training elsewhere in the European Union. It will no longer be satisfactory to have doctors training for between 8 and 12 years before achieving their consultant post, the average time-scale for training will move to 6 years. The recommendations of this report have been accepted by the government and are currently being implemented.

The changes planned include:

- the reduction in the duration of specialist training
- more structured and intensive training programmes
- the introduction of a unified training grade by amalgamating the registrar and senior registrar grades
- clear end-point to training with the award of a Certificate of Completion of Specialist Training.

These changes will result in a further reduction in the service contribution from medical staff in the training grades – thus compounding the problems from the reduction in junior doctors' hours. Clearly, these issues were instrumental in research such as the Greenhalgh Report (1994). This study, commissioned by the Department of Health, started from the premise that a number of everyday activities traditionally undertaken by junior doctors could be carried out by suitably trained nurses. The study was interested in finding out what work could be shared between junior doctors and nurses *for the benefit of patient care.* The six activities listed in Box 13.2 were identified as having the most potential for shared responsibility and demonstrated no statistical difference in quality when undertaken by a nurse (Greenhalgh Report 1994). The report estimates that between 11–16% (on days) and 12–24% (on nights) of junior doctors' time on wards is spent on these six activities all of which you will note are pertinent to day surgery nursing.

It is of note that the report emphasizes the need to *share* responsibility for these activities in the interests of improving the quality of life for junior doctors, improving communication and improving planning of care, rather than for them to be transferred wholesale to nurses; local

Box 13.2 Six activities able to be shared between doctors and nurses

1. Taking patient histories.
2. Venous blood sampling.
3. Insertion of peripheral intravenous (IV) cannulae.
4. Referring patients for investigations.
5. Writing discharge letters to GPs and other doctors.
6. IV drug administration, via peripheral cannulae (excluding cytotoxic drugs and first doses).

interpretations, however, do not always appear to make this explicit. Amongst the recommendations of the report there is a commitment to:

- a team-based approach to care
- all nurses undertaking the identified activities (with others considered at a local level)
- the activities becoming integral, rather than an extension, to the role of all nurses
- fostering collaborative practice and integrated patient records (see Chapter 6)
- inclusion of these six activities to competence level and experience in collaborative practice in all pre-registration nurse education programmes and undergraduate medical training.

Issues for Nursing and Professional Practice

The findings and recommendations of the Greenhalgh Report have been welcomed by many who see the opportunity to expand the nurse's role for the benefit of patient care. Equally, this report and the United Kingdom Central Council's position paper on 'The Scope of Professional Practice' (UKCC 1992) are viewed with some suspicion by others who foresee a dilution of nursing skills and see the transfer of some aspects of doctors' work as the thin end of the wedge. It is perhaps worth considering the two sides of this debate in relation to the future needs of patients in day surgery. A fundamental question appears to lie at the centre of the debate:

> Why do nurses appear dissatisfied with the essential caring nature of their role and seek therefore to 'develop' that role with aspects of doctors' work?

The Greenhalgh Report is at pains to point out that any sharing of responsibility is in the patients' best interests and should benefit care planning and quality of patient care. This is quite a seductive argument; many nurses will believe that taking on responsibility for certain procedures (especially it seems, the more technical ones) will ultimately benefit patient care as only they have full understanding of patients' needs and the skills to meet those needs. Unfortunately, as Hoover and van Ooijen (1995) point out, it would be quite easy to extend this argument to almost any aspect of medical care, an outcome clearly bordering on the ridiculous. Likewise, McAlister and Chiam (1995) describe as 'absurd' the commonly held belief that undertaking medical tasks somehow enhances the status of nurses and nursing.

However, this appears to be the route that some groups of nurses are eager to follow. Current nursing literature is replete with accounts of nurse surgical assistants (Tuthill 1995), nurse endoscopists (Gut Special Report 1995, Hughes 1996) and nurse anaesthetists (Carlisle 1996). Terms such as 'nurse practitioner' (Castledine 1993) and 'advanced practitioner' blur the picture, a situation further confused by the UKCC's lack of recognition of the specific roles, electing instead to define 'specialist' and 'advanced' levels of practice (Ford & Walsh 1994). But the lack of universally accepted definitions of these roles makes their evaluation difficult, if not impossible, with Read and George (1994) arguing that 'for nurse practitioner, read doctor substitution'. This view is not surprising as the role's origins are to be found in the USA; a response in the 1960s to a shortage of doctors and health care's rapidly rising costs (Ford & Walsh 1994). The title 'nurse practitioner' is a tautology; surely every practising nurse, by definition, can claim to be a nurse practitioner? Similar confusion is associated with the term 'theatre practitioner' – all qualified staff employed in theatres are theatre practitioners by definition; nurses and ODAs. Whilst Ford and Walsh (1994) argue that titles are less important than roles and responsibilities, research undertaken by Dowling *et al.* (1995) recognizes some of the ambiguities:

> The terms 'nurse practitioner' and 'nurse specialist' and other related titles may be used differently by hospitals for posts requiring varying levels of skill, roles and responsibilities.

This is an interesting study that is worth seeking out – an overview is found in Box 13.3.

Although only a very small percentage of the total number of practising nurses are following this route, the principle of behind such developments is worthy of question. Is *nursing* really so commonplace and limited that job satisfaction is only to be found in routinely undertaking specific aspects of a doctor's role without the associated career path, status or remuneration? Some appear to think so, and it is not too difficult to see the attraction of such posts to Trusts for day surgery and other areas in the future. But is this really what we want? We do want to develop specialist nurses in day surgery so that we can ensure strong clinical leadership, evidence-based practice and opportunities for consultancy, but not what Farmer (1995) describes as 'second-class doctors'. We do want flexible practitioners, able to support patients throughout their day surgery experiences, but not to the extent that they know a little of everything but are master of nothing. Morgan and Reynolds' study of the appeal of day surgery units to nurses in 1991 identified perceived status and career prospects as the least favoured aspects of working in day surgery. Nurses were 'concerned about the views of other nurses in the hospital', in that they thought their more social working hours were being equated with a lighter workload. But attempting to become a 'jack of all trades' is not the answer. We agree with Sutherland's (1994) concerns that 'multi-skilling' of nurses in day surgery in the mistaken belief that this enhances their status 'sells nurses and nursing short professionally' and can result in substandard care.

It is also of interest that this study highlighted the importance of primary nursing in day surgery units with the short but quite intensive relationship inherent in such a means of patient care delivery providing enormous job satisfaction. This involves a named nurse admitting their patients, preparing them for surgery, supporting them during induction of anaesthesia, helping them recover and providing postoperative care up to and including discharge and telephone follow-up. As West (1994) points out, the 'named nurse' concept, most easily achieved with a primary nursing system, is the most relevant aspect of the Patient's Charter for nurses, yet too frequently, for a host of reasons, nursing staff appear to be paying lip service to this important means of individualizing patient care. Photograph boards, coloured name badges and first name terms are no substitute for meaningful relationships based on trust (West 1994). Any 'multi-skilling' of day surgery nurses should therefore be in pursuit of greater continuity and quality of care for patients.

To conclude this discussion, consider the key points raised by Farmer (1995) in response to calls for interdisciplinary education (an editorial article well worth seeking out):

- 'the future of nursing is concerned with health and healing, not taking on jobs that doctors no longer want
- the roles of nurses and doctors are *not* interchangeable
- there is much to be gained from humanizing medicine but nothing to be gained from medicalizing nursing
- second-class doctoring is a poor substitute for first-class nursing' (Farmer 1995).

Box 13.3 Research Study

This exploratory study by Dowling *et al.*, carried out in 1993, sought to identify the professional, educational and management issues arising out of developing three nurses' roles to include aspects of medical practice. The authors recognize that traditional boundaries between the clinical work of junior doctors and nurses in the acute sector are being redrawn, with the reduction in junior doctors' hours and changes in specialist training being the key pressures for change. The researchers identify three major issues influencing the focus of the research:

- new roles should support patient care
- there is a need to respect educational, management and personal support needs of staff when taking on such new roles; i.e. change is not easy
- innovation and risk are respected.

For reasons identified above and to aid clarity, all three nurses involved in the fieldwork aspect of the study are referred to as postholders. Individual semi-structured interviews were conducted with stakeholders in the development – the nurse in post, junior doctors, consultants and other key staff with whom the postholder worked. Key issues explored were experiences of the new post and perceptions of its benefits and limitations. Two posts (A & B – in progress 9 and 18 months respectively) share many similarities and are discussed together. Post C (8 months' duration) is very different. All were paid the equivalent of clinical grades G or H.

- **Posts A** (gastroenterology) **& B** (urology and general surgery) are characterized by a short consultant-lead planning phase, driven by a new consultant appointment with no pre-registration house officer (HO) attached. **Nursing is specifically excluded from role definitions of both posts.** Postholders underwent very little preparation for the roles which involve, essentially, partial substitution of routine aspects of house officer work. Both nurses enjoyed their role. Major findings included:
- decreased HO workload, but no decrease in hours
- increased workload for senior house officers (SHO) and registrars
- no career path for nurses
- no associated nursing qualification gained
- concerns about possible deskilling of professional nurses
- postholders professionally isolated and vulnerable
- increased fragmentation of bedside care
- thought to be a quick solution
- low educational and management costs incurred in development.

Post C (neonatal) – a regionally funded post, patient care driven and several years in the planning. **This is an advanced nursing role** with almost total substitution of SHO clinical work with only tasks legally confined to medical practitioners, excluded. Major findings included:

- decreased workload and hours for SHOs
- training time made available for SHOs
- a small increase in workload for registrars
- a large increase in consultant teaching (to the postholder)
- a new career path in clinically advanced nursing
- promotion of clinical authority and professional autonomy
- associated transferable and validated advanced nursing qualification gained
- professionally and educationally supported
- high costs incurred in development
- potential for improved front line clinical care.

The authors conclude that the scope of new roles such as these is maximized when they are **an expansion of nursing**. They fear that if nurses continue to take on increasing amounts of medical and technical work, then valued characteristics of nursing may be threatened. There is a clear need for national and regional strategic planning and further research.

Summary

In this chapter we have attempted to raise several difficult issues being faced by the NHS, medical staff, nursing staff and the professions allied to medicine. We cannot predict what is going to happen over the next 5–10 years within the health service but the themes covered here will undoubtedly play a central part. In particular, the medical staffing and nursing and professional practice issues discussed will develop in parallel (each influencing the other) over this period. These more than anything else will be affected by the 'politics' of the decade and will play a major part in dictating the future shape of our specialty and the health service as a whole.

Key Points

- The development of free-standing day surgery centres on the lines of those in the USA with hotel beds close by may provide a lower cost alternative for some Trusts.
- Day surgery in general practitioner fundholding practices may increase in line with a move towards a primary health care led health service. Safety, economics and political will be the major determinants of its growth and success.
- The provision of hotel services, staffed by reception and catering personnel on Trust premises offers the possibility of more complex surgery being undertaken at a lower cost than an overnight stay in hospital.
- Minimal access surgical techniques will continue to develop.
- New anaesthetic techniques allow for even greater precision in administration and facilitating safer anaesthesia for patients.
- Current shortage of anaesthetists limits provision of anaesthetic services to peripheral units and requires optimal use of staff in post.
- Roles such as surgical assistants and nurse endoscopists are likely to grow in response to changes in medical training and reductions in junior doctors' hours, but must not compromise patient care.
- Nursing as a profession must safeguard the valued characteristics of nursing and develop new roles that are an expansion of nursing.
- Day surgery needs strong clinical leadership and evidence-based practice, not 'second-class doctors' (Farmer 1995).

Recommended Reading

Fowler, C. (1994) **The future of minimal access surgery.** *British Journal of Theatre Nursing* **4**(10): 5–6

A part tongue-in-cheek view of one possible 'minimal access' future

Dowling, S., Barrett, S. and West, R. (1995) **With nurse practitioners, who needs house officers?** *British Medical Journal* **311**: 309–313

A relevant and readable research study exploring the development of nursing roles

Farmer, E. (1995) **Medicine & nursing: a marriage for the 21st century?** *British Journal of Nursing* **4**(14): 793–794

An incisive and insightful perspective on increasing the technical and medical aspects of nursing

References

The Allitt Inquiry (the Clothier Report) (1994) **Report of the independent inquiry relating to deaths and injuries on the children's ward at Grantham and Kesteven General Hospital during the period of February to April 1991.** London: HMSO.

Association of Anaesthetists (1995) **Surgery and General Anaesthesia in General Practitioner Premises.** Association of Anaesthetists.

Baggott, R. (1994) **Health & Health Care in Britain.** Basingstoke: Macmillan.

Bloor, K. and Maynard, A. (1994) **Through the keyhole.** *The Health Service Journal* **104**(5429) 17 Nov: 24–26.

Carlisle, D. (1996) **Crossing the line.** *Nursing Times* **92**(23): 26–29.

Castledine, G. (1993) **Nurse Practitioner title: ambiguous and misleading.** *British Journal of Nursing* **2**(14): 734–735.

Department of Health (1991) **Welfare of children and young people in hospital.** London: HMSO.

Dowling, S., Barrett, S. and West, R. (1995) **With nurse practitioners, who needs house officers?** *British Medical Journal* **311**: 309–313.

Farmer, E. (1995) **Medicine & nursing: a marriage for the 21st century?** *British Journal of Nursing* **4**(14): 793–794.

Ford, P. and Walsh M. (1994) **New Rituals for Old. Nursing through the Looking Glass.** Oxford: Butterworth–Heinemann.

Greenhalgh Report (1994) **The interface between junior doctors and nurses: A research study for the Department of Health.** Macclesfield: Greenhalgh & Company.

Gut Special Report (1995) **The nurse endoscopist.** *Gut* **36**: 795.

Hoover, J. and van Ooijen, E. (1995) **Back to basics.** *Nursing Times* **92**(33): 42–43.

Hughes, M. (1996) **Key issues in the introduction of nurse endoscopy.** *Nursing Times* **92**(8): 38–39.

MacAlister, L. and Chiam, M. (1995) **Why do nurses agree to take on doctors' roles?** *British Journal of Nursing* **4**(21): 1238–1239.

Morgan, M. and Reynolds, A. (1991) **Day surgery units: Are they attractive to nurses?** *Journal of Advances in Health and Nursing Care* **1**(2): 59–74.

NATN (1995) **Operating Department Practitioners, NVQ Level 3: the new updated standards. A statement from NATN.** *British Journal of Theatre Nursing* **5**(7): 10–11.

NHS Management Executive (1991) **Junior doctors: The new deal.** London: NHS ME.

Philips, K. (1994) **Minimally invasive surgery.** *British Journal of Theatre Nursing* **3**(12): 4–8.

Read, S. and George, S. (1994) **Nurse Practitioners in A&E departments; reflections on a pilot study.** *Journal of Advanced Nursing* **19**: 705–716.

Royal College of Anaesthetists and the College of Ophthalmologists (1993) **Report of the joint working party on anaesthesia in ophthalmic surgery.** Royal College of Anaesthetists and the College of Ophthalmologists.

Sutherland, R. (1994) **Is this the way forward?** *British Journal of Theatre Nursing* **4**(1): 12–13.

Thornes, R. (1991) **Just for the day – Caring for children in the health services.** London: NAWCH.

Tuthill, V. (1995) **The training of nurse surgical assistants.** *British Journal of Nursing* **4**(21): 1240–1245.

United Kingdom Central Council for Nursing, Midwifery & Health Visiting (1992) **The scope of professional practice.** London: UKCC.

West, B. J. M. (1994) **Named nursing – a forced choice?** *Surgical Nurse* **7**(3): 4–5.

Working Group on Specialist Medical Training (Calman Report) (1993) **Hospital doctors: Training for the future.** London: DoH.

Index

Numbers in *italics* refer to illustrations or tables